Advanced Family Work for Schizophrenia

Advanced Family Work for Schizophrenia

An evidence-based approach

Julian Leff

Gaskell

© The Royal College of Psychiatrists 2005

Gaskell is an imprint of the Royal College of Psychiatrists, 17 Belgrave Square, London SW1X 8PG
http://www.rcpsych.ac.uk

British Library Cataloguing-in-Publication Data.
A catalogue record for this book is available from the British Library.
ISBN 1-904671-27-6

Distributed in North America by Balogh International Inc.

The Royal College of Psychiatrists is a registered charity (no. 228636).
Printed by Bell & Bain Limited, Glasgow, UK.

Contents

The author   vi

Acknowledgements   vii

1   Introduction   1

2   Culture clash   4

3   People with a psychotic illness and a physical condition   20

4   More than one family member with a psychosis   39

5   Parents in a conflictual relationship or separated   64

6   Dysfunctional families   77

7   Unresolved past trauma   86

8   Exploitative carer   91

9   Postscript   94

References   96

Index   99

The author

Julian Leff is Emeritus Professor at the Institute of Psychiatry, King's College London, and the Department of Mental Health Sciences, Royal Free and University College Medical School.

Acknowledgements

I am deeply indebted to Catherine Gamble, who attended the first training course we ran on family work for schizophrenia and emerged as one of the star pupils. She went on to become an internationally recognised trainer herself and has gained extensive experience both in working with families and in teaching others to do so. She read a draft of this book and made many instructive and constructive comments, which have been acted on to produce the final draft.

CHAPTER 1

Introduction

In 1976 my colleagues and I began to develop an approach to working with the families of people with schizophrenia. This was a joint effort in which a number of individuals collaborated over a period of about 10 years. They comprised professionals from several disciplines with differing theoretical orientations and training experiences. The key people were Elizabeth Kuipers, David Sturgeon, Rosemarie Eberlein-Fries, Ruth Berkowitz, Dominic Lam and Naomi Shavit. After completing two randomised controlled trials of the family work (Leff *et al*, 1982, 1985, 1989, 1990), we began training community psychiatric nurses in the techniques and learned more about the essential skills we needed to teach. These experiences culminated in a book *Family Work for Schizophrenia* by Elizabeth Kuipers, myself and Dominic Lam, published in 1992. Accumulating experience and feedback on the first edition from colleagues led to the production of an expanded second edition in 2002.

For the past 10 years I have been supervising clinical teams in north and south London for family work. In most of the families discussed in these sessions the patients have a diagnosis of schizophrenia, but there have also been those with manic-depressive psychosis and a few with other psychiatric conditions. In addition, I have given ongoing supervision to overseas trainees who have attended a 2-week course run annually. This supervision has mainly involved trainees from Europe. As they gain experience, family workers learn to cope with the common problems presented by families doing their best to help a relative with a psychotic illness. Consequently the families they tend to present to a supervisor have particularly difficult problems. The need to help supervisees find ways of managing these problems stimulated me to think creatively about them, and also to ask the groups to brainstorm, since several heads are better than one.

Over time I came to realise that the manual we wrote needed supplementing with a text that provided guidance on issues such as psychiatric illness in more than one family member, patients with a combination of psychiatric and physical conditions or with dual diagnosis disorder, families in which members belong to different ethnic groups, and other complexities. Since a person with schizophrenia has approximately a 10% chance of having a parent with the same illness and a similar risk of having an affected sibling, multiply affected families are not uncommon. Furthermore, families of mixed ethnicity are on the increase as societies become progressively more multicultural. Hence family workers are likely to encounter such challenges to their skill and ingenuity fairly frequently.

In preparation for this book I reviewed the extensive notes I have kept about the families presented to me in supervision sessions, numbering over 150. From these I have selected 19 that illustrate the problems I consider to be most salient and instructive. I was keen to have feedback from the clinicians about their work with the families discussed in supervision sessions, to learn whether the suggested approaches had been successful, and if not, to discuss other ways of helping the families move forward. However, this was not always forthcoming, either because the family worker was not present at some of the supervision sessions or because the family failed to engage with ongoing work. In some instances families and the therapists working with them reach a plateau; that is, they advance to a certain stage and then seem to lose their impetus. This can happen when symptoms subside and there is a return to a more normal state. Everyone breathes a sigh of relief, failing to recognise that the work needs to enter a new phase, focusing on obtaining employment, promoting and sustaining outside relationships and enhancing the person's self-esteem. As a result of these eventualities, follow-up of the families described here ranges from 3 to 30 months, with an average of 12 months.

The problems represented by these illustrative families have been grouped under a small number of headings for ease of reference, but some of the families fall into more than one category. Although the case studies are based on real families, they are essentially fictional since not only have the names of family members and patients been changed but other personal and circumstantial details have been altered substantially, so that no family will be identifiable from these accounts. It should also be noted that I was not personally involved in the immediate care of any of these families and never met any member of them.

The supervisees represented all the disciplines included in community mental health teams: psychiatric nurses, psychologists, psychiatrists, social workers, occupational therapists and psychiatric assistants. Prior to attending the supervision sessions, very few had received any specific training in working with families caring for a relative with a psychotic illness. Although the rest may have met with family carers in the course of their work, none was equipped with the relevant skills to tackle the difficult problems encountered in these families. Central to the process of supervision was the use of role-play. Usually the person presenting the family would be asked to play one of the key family members. Other supervisees would play additional family members and the therapists. Role-play enables the rehearsal of suggested interventions and gives the group the opportunity to comment on the therapists' techniques and the family interactions, and to suggest alternative interventions.

The term 'therapist' is used in the text to refer to whichever professional was engaged in working with the families. I do not refer to family work as therapy since the family members are not considered to be in need of treatment. Rather they need to be seen as allies in the struggle to help the ill person recover from schizophrenia and fulfil their potential. However, the term 'therapist' is useful shorthand for referring to the many different professionals engaged in the family work. The supervisor referred to throughout was myself. I am very grateful to the supervisees who, over the years, have brought so many families' stories to our sessions together, enriching our experience and challenging us to find creative ways of easing the burdens of patients and their family carers.

CHAPTER 2

Culture clash

The 20th century was an era of the greatest migration of people, partly because of the two world wars and partly the relative ease of transcontinental travel. When migrant groups come into contact with the host culture there are a number of ways in which they can attempt to accommodate to the situation. One way is to strive to preserve their traditional cultural values and traditions, as seen in the Asian communities in the UK. Cohesive groups of this kind, intent on maintaining their cultural identity, strongly discourage intimate relationships with people from other cultures. Nevertheless, youngsters of the second generation may fall in love and form long-term relationships with those from different cultures. Problems can arise when one of the partners, or one or more of their children, suffer from a serious mental illness. This is not uncommon, particularly when one of the family members is of African or African–Caribbean descent, since these groups have an incidence of serious mental illness six to seven times that of the native White population (Fearon *et al*, 2004; Lloyd *et al*, 2005).

The problems differ according to the generation to which the patients belong. The host culture generally offers the attractions of a more affluent lifestyle and higher status. Second-generation migrants usually master the host's language, and many aspire to become part of the dominant culture. However, members of the host culture often reject the advances of second-generation migrants, particularly if they are identifiable by their skin colour. Of course there are exceptions, although even when long-term inter-cultural relationships are formed, ethnic differences between the partners can lead to a devaluing of the religious or cultural beliefs of one partner by the other. Partners can often have different concepts of mental illness, with one accepting a biomedical explanation and the resultant treatment and the other rejecting both diagnosis and treatment, adhering to a traditional view of the nature and causes of psychiatric illnesses. Disagreements may also arise over lifestyles and the respective roles of men and women in the family. In general, traditional family structure involves dominance of men over women, and rigid differentiation of roles and responsibilities. The 'new man' is a Western concept that has hardly touched the lifestyles of non-Western families.

Derogatory attitudes of the partner to the patient's religious or cultural beliefs can further lower the patient's self-esteem. Interventions are aimed at modelling and encouraging tolerance for the other's culture and/or religion. It can be helpful for patients to pursue an activity that is valued by their own cultural group. This not only offers them the opportunity to strengthen their identity but provides them with a support network from their own culture. In working with these families, therapists have to be very sensitive to cultural norms regarding communication; for example, in some traditional families dialogue between senior and junior members is restricted by hierarchical rules. Also, the concept of a private consultation is foreign to traditional cultures, and the family will expect to be present when a therapist sees the patient. This is fine for those embarking on work with the family, except that they need to be prepared for more people to be present than with the standard Western nuclear family. I have worked with families comprising two parents and four children, all of whom attended the family sessions.

Family 1. Leroy Hammond

History

Mr Hammond was born in Jamaica and immigrated to England at the age of 20, attracted by the promise of work. He soon found a job as a bus conductor and worked in this position for over 10 years. During the Brixton riots his manager made a racist remark in his presence, which he took personally and brooded over for some weeks. He began to believe that passers-by and passengers on his bus were insulting him. Eventually he accused a passenger of calling him a Black bastard and, in the course of the ensuing argument, hit him. He was referred to a psychiatrist and given a diagnosis of paranoid schizophrenia.

He responded reasonably well to treatment with an oral antipsychotic and was adherent to the medication for some years, managing to maintain his job on the buses. However, he then became involved with Rastafarianism, grew dreadlocks and began smoking cannabis regularly and frequently. Cannabis has the effect of intensifying his paranoid ideation, with the result that he becomes increasingly threatening and refuses to take his medication. He asserts that smoking cannabis is an essential tenet of his Rastafarian religion and has nothing to do with his illness. After a few years of repeated relapses he was discharged from his conductor's job on medical grounds.

His wife is 10 years younger than him and was born in Barbados. She is a practising Christian belonging to an evangelical church, and is derogatory about the Rastafarian religion, culture and music. She has become increasingly depressed and is critical of her husband's behaviour, his inability to work and his failure to take medication as prescribed.

There are three children of the marriage, one son and daughter who live away, and one daughter who lives at home and has a full-time job.

Presenting problems

Leroy is currently an in-patient, having recently experienced a relapse of his symptoms while on no medication. There have been acrimonious arguments at home between Leroy and his family over the medication. During an altercation with his son, Albert, both father and son were in tears. How can he be persuaded to take his medication and what can be done to deal with the family tensions?

Formulation

Many Caribbean men and women of working age were persuaded to migrate to the UK in the 1950s by a recruiting campaign in the West Indies. The majority of the immigrants found jobs in the newly established National Health Service, or, like Leroy, in the nationalised transport system. However, having a job and a better income than in their home countries did not satisfy their aspirations to be accepted as equal citizens by what was seen as the 'mother country'. Many African–Caribbeans encountered institutional racism in the police force, the judicial system and the government. The conservative government that was in power in the early 1960s enacted a series of immigration laws, which virtually put a stop to immigration from the 'New Commonwealth', including the West Indies. On a local level, signs in boarding houses proclaimed 'No children, no dogs, no coloureds'. African–Caribbean children were also actively discouraged from forming relationships with Whites and vice versa.

Furthermore, the second generation of African–Caribbeans fared far worse than their parents in the job market. The success of the recruiting campaign and the post-war baby boom provided the adults needed to make up the staffing shortages. Unemployment among African–Caribbeans born in the UK reached levels greatly in excess of their White counterparts. Leroy's children were fortunate to find jobs, but the general feeling of being disadvantaged and discriminated against pervaded the African–Caribbean community and became manifest in the Brixton riots. The racist remark by Leroy's manager might have had less impact on him at another time, but in this period of unrest it brought to a head Leroy's feeling of belonging to a persecuted minority. His paranoid ideation increasingly coloured his perceptions and culminated in an assault on a passenger, who was probably innocent of any derogatory remarks (Chadwick, 1995).

Caribbeans like Leroy who expected to be treated like Britishers, but who instead met with hostility and rejection, needed to establish an alternative identity of which they could feel proud. Leroy met this need by joining the Rastafarian movement/religion, but his wife Winsome found an accepting group of people in the Black evangelical church she attended. Unfortunately she was antagonistic to Leroy's choice of a group he could identify with, probably because of her religious convictions. Furthermore, the insistence by Rastafarians that smoking cannabis is part of their religious practice conflicts with Leroy's need to avoid it because of his psychiatric condition.

Although the Rastafarian group provides Leroy with support and enhances his sense of identity, it cannot compensate for his loss of a role as a working man and a provider for his family. This loss and the diagnosis of a serious mental illness are both blows to his pride and self-esteem.

Supervisor's suggestions

1. Negotiate with family members and convene a meeting with them all. *Rationale* The children are involved with their parents and can contribute a different perspective from their mother on the problems. They also have the potential to provide emotional support to both Leroy and Winsome.
2. To ensure that the engagement process continues smoothly, positive reframing techniques can be used; that is, negative attitudes to the patient are represented in a positive light. For example, anger stems from the fact that the relative cares about the patient. Consequently, stress the positive feelings of the family towards Leroy. Point out that the fact that father and son were both moved to tears by their disagreement shows that they have a deep concern for each other.
3. Focus on the sense of loss of each member. Leroy has lost his roles as a worker and breadwinner. Make the link between Leroy's loss of status and his aggression. The other family members have lost the husband and father they used to know. Winsome has lost the companionship of her partner and has become depressed. A high proportion of carers of people with schizophrenia develop sufficient symptoms of depression and anxiety to be in need of treatment (Singleton *et al*, 2002). Help the family to mourn these losses together and to give each other support in the process.
4. Ask Leroy and Winsome to explain to the others what they each appreciate about their religious affiliation. Encourage mutual respect for their choices.

5. Ask Winsome to tell Leroy one thing he could do to help or support her around the home. This was arguably a long shot because the traditional Caribbean male views housework as the woman's domain. This is an example of cultural values overriding the therapist's strategy.

Follow-up

There was no follow-up report for 8 months and then the therapist recounted what had happened in the intervening period. Leroy was discharged from the hospital after a few weeks and returned home. Shortly after, a family meeting was held which both parents and the three children attended. The therapist introduced the theme of loss and the family responded with a genuine feeling of sadness, particularly Winsome.

In subsequent sessions, not all of which were attended by the children, the therapist explored the benefits Leroy and Winsome derived from the religious groups to which they were affiliated. Winsome began to appreciate her husband's need to have a peer group that valued his contribution. When Winsome was asked what Leroy could do at home to help her she did not mention any assistance with the housework but requested that he refrained from smoking cannabis. He stated again that this was part of his religion and under no circumstances would he give it up. However, after some negotiation he agreed that he would not smoke it in their home, and this promise satisfied Winsome.

The therapist explored the possibility that Leroy might attend a day centre exclusively for Black patients, which provided activities he might enjoy. He agreed to visit it and was impressed with what was on offer. He began to attend regularly and became a member of the band, playing a steel drum. He also joined a creative writing class and wrote about his childhood in Jamaica and his experiences on coming to England.

At the time of the follow-up report, Leroy was taking antipsychotic medication regularly and was free of symptoms. Winsome was less depressed and their relationship had improved.

Commentary

Leroy had benefited from his children's expression of love and support, which helped to boost his self-esteem. Through getting the parents to explain what each valued about their religious affiliation, Winsome realised her husband's need to belong to a male peer group that gave him a sense of pride. The Black day centre provided Leroy with an alternative support group (to the Rastafarians), in which his creative talents found expression. Writing about his childhood and the negative aspects of his life in England enabled him to process the losses he had sustained and to recognise the commonality of his experiences with others in the day centre. His agreement not to smoke cannabis at home and his adherence to the prescribed medication improved the relationship with his wife. As a result she was better able to fulfil her role as carer and her depression receded.

Family 2. Charlene Ogunseke

History

Charlene is 33 years old and is married with three children. She was born in Jamaica and lived there until the age of 6. Her parents then immigrated to England, bringing Charlene and her two sisters with them. Charlene experienced sexual abuse from her father from the age of 11 to 13. She eventually told her mother who alerted the authorities. Her father was imprisoned and her mother took the children to live in another part of the city. The mother worked as the manager of a laundrette.

Charlene did well at school and left at age 18, finding a job as a legal secretary for 6 years. She then became pregnant and her mother sent her back to Jamaica to stay with an aunt. This was in order to conceal her illegitimate pregnancy from relatives and friends in England. For this reason, when the baby was born her mother persuaded Charlene to leave the child in Jamaica and return to England. Her mother has since retired and has returned to Jamaica for good.

On returning, Charlene worked in casual jobs as a typist. She married at age 26 a Nigerian student named Tolani Ogunseke. At first she did not tell her husband about her child in Jamaica, but revealed this later. She gave birth to two daughters, both of whom are now attending primary school. She fell pregnant 3 months after the birth of the second daughter and became increasingly distressed during the pregnancy. Following the birth she became psychotic and was admitted for several weeks. An initial diagnosis was made of puerperal psychosis, but subsequently she has had three brief admissions for episodes of psychosis unrelated to pregnancy and the diagnosis has been revised to schizophrenia. One of her sisters suffers from schizophrenia, but they have no contact as her family in England disapprove of her husband.

Charlene is on a monthly depot injection of an antipsychotic and adheres well to the treatment. Nevertheless she experiences continuous auditory hallucinations. She has learned to cope with these by ignoring them.

Tolani is a perpetual student and is coming to the end of a social sciences course. He also works as a volunteer for a mental health organisation. He and Charlene were living in a council flat that was in his name. However, on discharge from the mother and baby unit after recovering from her first episode of psychosis, she refused to return to the council flat. They were rehoused in a garden flat and she was awarded sickness benefit. She attends a women's group in a day centre weekly and also goes to a cookery class, but is very passive and only socialises through the church she attends. Tolani wants her to enrol in a course of study with the aim of going to a university.

Tolani is very critical of her. He complains that she is lazy, neglects her appearance and doesn't cope with the housework. She allows him to do the housework because he is so critical of what she does. Although it is unusual in his culture of origin for men to do housework, he explained that he was brought up in a female household and took on many female roles. Charlene takes the children to school. Tolani buys her clothes for her and controls most aspects of her life. Despite his criticisms he wants to stay with her. They have had no sexual relations since the birth of her last child.

Presenting problems

It is difficult to work with Tolani because he does not accept a medical explanation for his wife's problems, but asserts that she is not ill. The therapist noticed bottles of whisky and wine in the home and Tolani stated that Charlene had had a drinking problem for at least 3 years. Husband and wife argue all the time over her drinking. He has been hitting her and she came to the day centre with a black eye. He wants her to get treatment for the drinking and go to college. How can the relationship between the couple be improved? What can be done about Charlene's drinking?

How can Tolani be persuaded to have more realistic expectations for his wife?

Formulation

Black people have been migrating to the UK for several centuries. The big influx of African–Caribbeans occurred between 1950 and 1962. People from Africa have been coming in increasing numbers in the past few decades, mostly for different reasons from the African–Caribbeans. Some have been escaping the civil wars and massacres in African countries, notably in the Sudan and Somalia. Others are intent on studying and obtaining prestigious British qualifications, as in Tolani's case. The attitude towards study differs markedly between the two Black immigrant groups. Whereas the African students view living in Britain as a great opportunity to improve their academic status, African–Caribbeans are suspicious of a life devoted to study, seeing excessive study ('studiation') as leading to mental disorders (Littlewood, 1988). Hence it is not surprising that Charlene resists the pressure from Tolani to take on a course of study.

It is an error to equate African cultures with the cultures in the Caribbean. Although the Africans forced into slavery and transported to the West Indies took their cultures with them, three centuries of living under the domination of slave owners who deliberately tried to destroy their cultural roots inevitably had a major impact. Furthermore, each of the Caribbean islands developed its own local culture coloured by the language and customs of the dominant groups. Therefore there is a considerable disparity between Charlene's cultural background in Jamaica and Tolani's in Nigeria.

The sexual abuse that Charlene suffered from her father in childhood continues to have an effect on her life. Recent studies have identified childhood sexual abuse as a risk factor for auditory hallucinations (Hammersley *et al*, 2003; Janssen *et al*, 2004), and continuous auditory hallucinations are the most prominent feature of Charlene's illness.

The other major life event was her first, illegitimate pregnancy and the way in which her mother handled it, inducing in her a sense of shame. It is likely that this influenced her attitude to her subsequent two pregnancies with Tolani. The fact that she fell pregnant again so soon after the birth of her second child with Tolani clearly distressed her and may have been a major factor in her post-partum psychosis. Her refusal to have sexual relations with her husband is obviously related to both the unwanted third pregnancy with Tolani and the development of her mental illness following the birth.

In terms of expressed emotion, Tolani is critical of his wife and also hostile, since he calls her lazy, failing to understand that her inertia is a result of her illness; he has physically abused her. He is also overinvolved as shown by his taking over her roles in the care of the house and the children, and the degree of control he exerts over her life. Over-involvement is not common among spouses, nor does it usually coexist with hostility, although criticism is quite often voiced by overinvolved relatives (Leff and Vaughn, 1985). The combination of negative emotions expressed by Tolani is evocative of the concept of the double bind (Bateson *et al*, 1956). In essence he is saying to Charlene 'I don't like what you do and who you are, but I am not going to let you get away from me.'

Charlene has lost nearly all her valued roles. She is no longer able to sustain a paid job, she cannot be a mother to her first child and her mothering of the other three children has been eroded by Tolani. She cannot act as a daughter to her mother, who has returned to Jamaica, nor to her father from whom she is alienated. Her role as a wife has been undermined by the cessation of sexual relations with her husband. All that is left is her role as a sick person, which it is therefore difficult for her to relinquish. Her drinking is an expression of her sense of loss of what she could have achieved without her devastating life experiences and the emotional and psychological disturbances that followed.

Supervisor's suggestions

1. Her drinking problem needs to be addressed by referral to a specialist service since it is provoking physical abuse by her husband. However, the psychological reasons for her drinking must not be neglected. Dual diagnosis often poses significant challenges for all concerned. Traditionally substance misuse has been thought of as a specialist area, but there is now growing acceptance that all practitioners need to have knowledge and skills in working with this problem, since people with these difficulties have higher rates of suicide, homelessness, violence, non-adherence to medication and relapse (Department of Health, 2002).

2. The sexual abuse she suffered as a child is still exerting an effect on her and she is now experiencing physical abuse from her husband. She is receiving some support from the women's group she attends, but she also needs to join a group for survivors of sexual abuse.

3. She must be helped to strengthen her roles as a mother and as a wage-earner. The former requires work with Tolani to reduce his overprotective, controlling behaviour. The latter might be achieved by attendance at a rehabilitation service. In view of her premorbid work history, it is likely that she could cope with a part-time job in open employment.

4. She has developed a strategy to manage her persistent auditory hallucinations, but she might benefit from learning about other coping methods by joining a 'hearing voices' group. This should also help her to feel less of an outsider.

5. Attempts should be made to heal the rift with her relatives in her locality. She has a very limited social network and could gain from the additional support her family could provide. Contact with her sister who also suffers from schizophrenia might make her feel less uniquely abnormal.

6. Education about schizophrenia should be given to Tolani and Charlene together, with the aim of reducing his critical attitude towards her. In these sessions she should be regarded as the expert and encouraged to describe her auditory hallucinations in the hope that he might appreciate the nature of her experiences and illness. A strong emphasis is needed on the effect of schizophrenia in sapping energy and interest.

7. Tolani's overinvolvement can be addressed by focusing on his need to control so much of Charlene's life and exploring what he fears would happen if he gave her more freedom. He should be encouraged to devote more of his time to his voluntary work with the mentally ill, as an alternative outlet for his caring needs.

8. When the therapist has gained the confidence of both partners, the issue of their lack of sexual relations should be raised. In particular,

Charlene's anxieties about becoming pregnant again need to be openly discussed.

Follow-up

2 months

She was referred to a survivors' group and made good use of it to express her grief and anger at her father's abuse of her, but also her guilt at instigating his imprisonment. She was also referred to an alcohol service, which she attended twice and was then discharged. Her excessive drinking has settled down. It seems that her husband may have exaggerated the problem.

A joint meeting was held with the couple in which information about schizophrenia was given. Charlene was encouraged to describe the voices she was hearing and how frequently they occur. Tolani was surprised by this account since she had concealed the experiences from him. He was able to appreciate that they were caused by a mental illness, but could not accept that her self-neglect and slowness were anything other than laziness. It was explained to them both that Charlene needed further training to enable her overcome these problems and to get back to paid work. He was pleased with this suggestion because it was in accordance with his aim for her to attend an educational course.

4 months

She made contact with her sister and met her once, but found her to be much more disabled by her illness than she is and was reluctant to continue seeing her. She also refused to consider joining a 'hearing voices' group as she felt it would distress her to focus on her voices. It is relatively common for people who have experienced an episode of psychosis to seal it over and put it behind them. Professionals, who prefer their patients to develop good insight, view this strategy negatively, but recent research has shown that sealing over is associated with a higher level of self-esteem than full insight (Morgan, 2003).

Charlene had begun to attend a rehabilitation course and was doing well. Tolani was attending college 3 days a week and was looking after the children up to 09.00 h. This enabled Charlene to take on a cleaning job for 2 h every morning.

A sudden change in their relationship occurred which provoked a major upheaval in their pattern of life. Tolani began sleeping away from home and stopped looking after the children. This forced her to cease attending the rehabilitation course and to give up the cleaning job. Although Tolani has distanced himself from her, he continues to do the shopping. She does the cooking and cleaning of the home. She looks after the children well and has a group of friends.

Commentary

The intervention of the therapist had the unexpected effect of producing a greater separation between Charlene and her husband. In retrospect there were two indications of this outcome: Tolani's hostility towards her, which often signifies a desire to be rid of the caring role, and the lack of any sexual intimacy between them. It is likely that he had found another sexual partner but still felt some responsibility for his family. His leaving home may also have been provoked by his recognition that Charlene had a serious mental illness, a fact that previously he had denied.

Attendance at the survivors' group and the rehabilitation course empowered Charlene to reclaim the roles that she had abandoned as a result of her illness and Tolani's overprotectiveness. His withdrawal freed her to develop her potential as a mother and as a social being, since she gained a circle of friends.

When faced with a poor marital relationship between clients, the therapist has no authority to decide what the preferred outcome should be. Instead the aim is to assist the partners to move towards their own decision. In this case the husband made a unilateral decision without any negotiation with his wife. It has certainly had positive effects on Charlene, but at this early stage it is too soon to predict the long-term consequences. The therapist needs to be in contact with her for the foreseeable future.

Family 3. Patience Adebole

History

Patience is aged 35. She emigrated from Nigeria at the age of 20 to study business administration and graduated 4 years later. During her studies she met her current partner, Moses Ebigbo, also from Nigeria, and they have lived together for 12 years. Moses used to run his own business but ran into financial problems and had to sell it. He is now employed by a computer company and works extremely long hours (over 12 h a day).

They have a son aged 10 and two daughters aged 8 and 5. Patience first developed schizophrenia 1 year after her last child was born. At that time she was working full time in a confectionary business, the children being cared for by a childminder. Her illness was characterised by religious and paranoid delusions. She heard voices that she identified as coming from her heart, telling her to leave the house and family. They made her feel shaky and hopeless. She believes the voices are dark forces. Her grandmother suffered from a similar illness. Patience has been admitted to hospital twice, the last occasion being during the previous year. She responded well to initial treatment with sulpiride but was opposed to taking medication and did not adhere to treatment. The medication was replaced by trifluoperazine in the hope of persuading her to take it regularly, but unfortunately she developed an oculogyric crisis, which reinforced her negative attitude to drugs. Recently her regimen was changed to a depot neuroleptic every 2 weeks, but she often refuses to accept the injection.

Patience attends an Apostolic church and has told members of the congregation of her problem. She reports that her pastor tells her not to take medication. Her mother in Nigeria, who is also devout, prays for her. When she is admitted to hospital Moses takes time off work to look after the children. He has a reasonable level of understanding of the illness and believes that Patience needs medication. He is supportive of her, but when she won't take medication he says she can pack her bags and go.

Presenting problems

Together with a colleague, the therapist has given education about schizophrenia to the couple. In an individual session, Patience confided in the therapist that she committed adultery some years previously while living with Moses. She has never told her partner this. In her first psychotic episode she saw messages on television referring to her infidelity. Should she be encouraged to tell Moses about this in order to relieve her feelings of guilt? How can she be persuaded to take the medication regularly?

Formulation

Patience is well-educated and in many ways Westernised. However, her antagonism to medication appears to stem from the beliefs of the religious group from which she receives valuable support. Her partner Moses is not a church-goer and accepts the biomedical explanation of her illness. The difference in their attitudes to medication is a source of serious conflict. The therapist would need to contact the pastor to discuss the importance of medication for Patience's health.

It is also possible that she is very sensitive to the side-effects of antipsychotic medication. In particular, a high proportion of patients experience sexual side-effects, such as impotence in men and anorgasmia in women (National Schizophrenia Fellowship, 2000). Professionals rarely enquire about these, although they can cause friction between patients and their partners. Patience has been prescribed depot injections every 2 weeks, although the plasma level of a long-acting preparation remains steady for 4–6 weeks after the injection. Increasing the frequency to every 2 weeks has the effect of increasing the plasma level and hence the likelihood of side-effects. It would be advisable to space out Patience's injections to every 4 weeks, which might improve her adherence.

Patience continues to hear voices and has not developed any strategies to cope with this. A range of possible strategies that she might try needs to be explained to her.

Patience's single act of infidelity weighs heavily enough on her mind to enter into the content of her delusions during a psychotic episode. It is risky to encourage her to be open with Moses about it, since his response is unpredictable. His threat to leave her if she won't take medication may be simply a ploy to put pressure on her, but it might also reflect a deeper dissatisfaction with their relationship. An alternative confidante would be her pastor, although Patience would need to be assured of his silence on the matter.

The young children of a parent with a psychotic illness are very rarely considered in treatment plans, other than the issue of whether the patient is able to care for them adequately. But young children have to contend with the difficult problem of understanding their ill parent's behaviour. Why does mummy suddenly have to go to hospital and why does she seem different when she comes back? Why does she talk to somebody we can't see? Did we do something to make her go away? These are the kind of questions in children's minds, which they are rarely given the opportunity to voice. This important area for exploration is grossly neglected in the professional literature, with one or two exceptions (e.g. Cooklin, 2004). The well parent is often too bound up with their own distress and confusion to give appropriate help to their children. It is therefore incumbent on the therapist to pay attention to the children's need for understanding.

Supervisor's suggestions

1. Make contact with the pastor to assess his attitude to Patience's medication.
2. Explore the side-effects of her current medication, particularly on her sex life. Change the frequency of the injection to monthly instead of 2-weekly.
3. See Patience on her own to discuss with whom she would feel comfortable enough to disclose her infidelity.
4. Involve the children in family sessions. Use the children to reinforce Patience's positive self-esteem and to recount their experience of her when well and when ill, since this might persuade her to be more adherent to the medication.
5. Help her develop further strategies to cope with the persistent voices.

Follow-up

1 month

The therapist spoke to the pastor over the phone. He asserted that he had told Patience to take her doctor's advice. It is clear, therefore, that Patience had misreported her pastor's attitude in order to add his authority to her attitude towards medication.

Her depot injections have been changed to once a month. She is pleased but complains of drowsiness and shakiness due to the medication. She says she is tired of the illness and has been thinking of suicide. The voices are continuing to tell her to leave her job and go home, but when at home she feels useless. She was previously working in the local council housing department as a filing clerk. The therapist has advised working on short-term goals in order to achieve her long-term goal of returning to work. Moses is not exerting pressure on her to take a job. She needs 'grief work' around her losses. The therapist and a colleague will be working with her on this issue.

The therapist has talked to the couple about involving the children in sessions. Moses felt the youngest wouldn't understand. It has not been possible to arrange a family session so far because of his long working hours.

Patience had arranged to fly to Nigeria on the day following the supervision session for spiritual healing.

2 months

She remains in Nigeria. Her husband reports no problem.

3 months

She has returned from Nigeria. She reported that she showed the depot injection to a psychiatrist there who told her not to take it. Her parents gave her the same advice. This report needs to be treated with caution given her misrepresentation of her pastor's advice. While in Nigeria she received spiritual healing from a traditional healer. On her return she refused the depot injection. She is now mentally well.

The therapist raised the possibility of her talking about her infidelity either to the pastor or to Moses. She rejected both as possible confidantes, saying that she did not think about it any more.

She has started applying for jobs and has been offered a position in customer services in a shoe retailing business.

In view of Patience's vulnerability to stress, in discussion with the supervisee it was agreed that Patience was potentially being too ambitious; that is, attempting to look after the children, the household and hold down a full-time job. It was likely that this need to take on and be good at everything represented her attempt to counter her low self-esteem. The supervisee was advised to involve the two elder children in a session and to encourage them to say how much they appreciate her.

4 months

A family session with the two older children took place. The children were very loving to Patience and expressed how much they had missed her when she was in Nigeria. She promised them she would not go away again for so long. She told them that she had not been well but that she was now better. The therapist emphasised how much the children appreciated their mother, that she had a lot of love to give them and that at their age they still needed her to spend time with them, particularly as their father is away at work so much of the day.

The therapist also continued to see Patience individually. She has agreed to take a novel antipsychotic. She is still looking for a job, but now realises she should restrict herself to part-time work. She has not been hearing voices since returning from Nigeria.

5 months

Patience's mother is coming from Nigeria to help with the children. Moses says Patience is well and is encouraging her to work part-time. She is thinking of applying to the Post Office.

Commentary

Members of the public in developing countries are generally eclectic when dealing with health problems. They often consult traditional healers alongside Western biomedical practitioners (Swartz, 1998). It appeared at first that Patience's resistance to medication was based on her affiliation with a Christian Apostolic sect. However, her pastor denied telling her not to take medication. Her investment in a return air ticket to Nigeria in order to consult a traditional healer indicates a deep-seated belief in the effectiveness of this approach to sickness. She must have absorbed this belief during her childhood years in Nigeria and retained it throughout her years in the UK. It surfaced when she became disillusioned with the attempts of Western medicine to treat her psychiatric illness.

After her return to the UK she reported that she no longer heard the voices. This improvement cannot be attributed to antipsychotic drugs, since at this stage she was on no medication. It could have been a consequence of confiding in the therapist the story of her infidelity, which she had told no one before, and thus relieving her sense of guilt. Alternatively, the session with the traditional healer might have had a beneficial effect on her anxiety and through this she achieved relief from the auditory hallucinations.

In developing countries such as India, the shortage of psychiatric professionals means that only a small proportion of people with psychoses receive biomedical treatments. The rest are probably treated exclusively by traditional healers. Yet the outcome for schizophrenia in India is considerably better than in the West (Jablensky *et al*, 1992), suggesting that traditional treatments may have a therapeutic effect on the patients. Patience retained a belief in the value of traditional treatment and a scepticism about Western medicines, although it was reported in the last supervision session that she had agreed to take a novel antipsychotic. It is conceivable that she would be more adherent to this medication since it gives rise to fewer side-effects.

The meeting with her two older children enabled them to convey to her how much they loved her and needed her. Her response was to give them an explanation for her absences and to promise not to leave them for long periods again. This experience led to her modifying her unrealistic ambition to fulfil the roles of mother, homemaker and full-time wage earner. The conflict she felt between the pull of these different roles was expressed in the content of her auditory hallucinations. If she becomes more regular in taking her medication she may remain well, but resolving the conflict over her different roles is likely to strengthen her ability to deal with a further relapse if one occurs.

CHAPTER 3

People with a psychotic illness and a physical condition

The combination of psychosis and chronic physical disease poses difficult management problems for patients and their carers. Insulin-dependent diabetes, for example, requires strict adherence to a diet and to a medication regime. If there are already difficulties with adherence to an antipsychotic regime, these are exacerbated by the additional strictures of the treatment for diabetes. Furthermore, the weight gain caused by some antipsychotic drugs is antipathetic to the control of the diabetes and hypo- and hyperglycaemic episodes can complicate the psychiatric picture. The side-effect of weight gain is of particular significance to patients who have an eating disorder in addition to schizophrenia. It is noteworthy that one study has demonstrated a relationship between high expressed emotion in the carer and poor control of diabetes (Koenigsberg *et al*, 1993). Thus the outcome of both the psychiatric and the physical condition may be improved by family work.

It is not uncommon to encounter psychosis and learning difficulties in the same individual. When people with schizophrenia make a first contact with the psychiatric services their IQ is found to be between 87 and 89 on average. This suggests a drop in their IQ over the preceding period, which is supported by a falling-off in academic performance that often occurs in the early teenage years before the overt appearance of psychotic symptoms. We are not concerned with this phenomenon here but with learning difficulties that become evident in early childhood. The combination of learning difficulties with psychosis is particularly likely to engender overinvolved attitudes in carers: both family members and professionals. Mothers tend to become overprotective towards a young child with learning difficulties, although it may be difficult for an observer to judge what an appropriate level of protection should be. When a person with learning difficulties develops a psychotic illness, a mother with overinvolved attitudes is almost bound to intensify these.

Sensory defects in a person with a psychotic illness are particularly difficult to manage. Impairment of hearing or vision requires the care of specialists in these areas of medicine and cooperation by the patient in accepting remedial action. Paranoid delusions can be exacerbated if patients with impaired hearing fail to wear their hearing aid. Patients with impaired vision can endanger themselves or others if they do not heed professional advice concerning the precautions they need to take.

It is far from easy to achieve a smooth liaison between the various agencies dealing with the different aspects of the patient's well-being. Specialised services tend to be segregated from each other. Even bringing together a service for learning difficulties and one for psychosis can require considerable sustained efforts.

Family 4. Alicia Hammond

History

Alicia is aged 26 and has suffered from schizophrenia from the age of 12. Both her parents are from Jamaica but Alicia was born in the UK. At about the time Alicia's illness began, her father died, and her mother Marianne believes that Alicia is possessed by her father's spirit. She took Alicia to spiritual healers in Jamaica 2 years after she became ill to have the spirit exorcised.

Alicia's first admission was to a child psychiatry unit, following which Marianne took legal action to get her discharged. Alicia is overweight and has insulin-dependent diabetes and learning difficulties. During one psychotic episode she ran into the road and was injured by a car, which has left her with limited mobility.

As Alicia has difficulty managing her diabetes, a nurse comes daily to administer her insulin injection. Marianne has impaired vision and back trouble, and to assist her a home help was arranged, but she stopped the service after receiving a bill for it.

Marianne has two older children, Nelson who lives close by and attends a college of higher education, and Claire who lives with the family but who is studying maths at another college and spends little time at home. Marianne has at times locked Alicia in the house when she has gone out because she feels she cannot trust her to stay in on her own. Alicia eats indiscriminately and will take Claire's food. She spends a lot of time in bed.

Presenting problems

Mother can be quite antagonistic to the psychiatric services and has to be approached cautiously over every issue. She seems to be incapable of keeping Alicia to the recommended diet. She has blocked attempts to get Alicia to attend a day centre in the past on the grounds that she would not get the attention and understanding she needs. How can Alicia's physical health be safeguarded? How can she be encouraged to be more active and do more for herself?

Formulation

Alicia has three different sets of health problems: schizophrenia, learning difficulty and diabetes. Her learning difficulty has been present since birth and her other two conditions since childhood. It is not surprising, therefore, that her mother has developed overinvolved and overprotective attitudes. These are shown by Marianne removing Alicia from the child psychiatry unit, not wanting her to attend a day centre and locking her in the house on her own. She is antagonistic to the psychiatric services, an attitude commonly seen among overinvolved carers, who fear the professionals will displace them from their valued role. Consequently they denigrate the services offered and question the competence of the professional carers. The therapist felt she had to be very cautious in the suggestions she proposed for fear of antagonising Marianne.

There is an additional complication arising from Marianne's belief that her daughter is, or was, possessed by her dead father's spirit. This could lead her to reject biomedical explanations of Alicia's mental problems. This belief is consonant with Marianne's cultural upbringing in Jamaica (see Family 1). It is vital to avoid conflict with carers over explanations for a psychiatric illness in a family member. The therapist can state that there are many different ways of explaining these illnesses and that it is most helpful for the patient when each party respects the preferred explanation of the other.

The therapist has to be extremely careful to avoid the carer feeling that they are being criticised and displaced from their role. It is essential to recognise that overinvolved carers are doing what they believe to be best for the patient, and are devoting a huge amount of time and energy to this task, which has often become the centre of their lives. The first step in defusing the carer's suspicion of professional intervention is to congratulate them on the care they are giving their relative and express awareness of how much time and energy it takes. Once the therapist has reassured the carer, they can proceed to discuss how the carer can help their relative to become more independent. It is important not to exclude the carer from this endeavour or they will sabotage it. In this instance Marianne could be asked to accompany Alicia to the day centre for a trial visit and to help her choose a suitable activity that she might enjoy.

It was discovered a long time ago that carers respond more normally when asked about their healthy children than when the enquiry is about the child with mental illness (Sharan, 1966). Consequently Marianne should be congratulated on bringing up two such successful people as Nelson and Claire, latterly without the help of a husband. The children should be invited to at least one family meeting for a number of reasons.

Healthy children, particularly those who have successfully achieved independence, are often able to be objective about the family situation and to make perceptive observations in direct language. They may be induced to share some of the caring tasks, thus reducing the burden on the primary carer. They may also be able to help the patient socialise with an age-appropriate peer group.

Alicia's triple health problems require close coordination between the different services involved. It is often difficult to achieve a good working relationship between services for adult mental illness and for learning difficulties. Commonly each service would like to shift the whole responsibility for the patient to the other. It becomes even more complicated to manage when a service for physical illness is also involved, as in Alicia's case. It is most helpful to convene a joint meeting between representatives of all the relevant services with the aim of agreeing on a rational management strategy. Alicia's overeating may stem from her learning difficulty, or her schizophrenia, or may be an independent eating disorder. Whatever its origin it is inimical to control of her diabetes, and illustrates the necessity for communication and coordination between the three services. It is advisable that Marianne be invited to attend this meeting as an active participant, since if she feels excluded from the decisions, she is likely to sabotage whatever plan is agreed upon and to set one service against the other.

Supervisor's suggestions

1. Meet with Marianne and Alicia and congratulate mother on the fulfilling of her caring role. Suggest that mother takes Alicia to the day centre and helps her choose an appropriate activity.
2. Invite the healthy brother and sister to a family meeting and ask them each to suggest one thing they could do to help Alicia.
3. Organise a meeting of all the professionals involved in Alicia's care and include Marianne.

Follow-up

1 month

The therapist saw mother and Alicia together. Mother talked for Alicia all the time and did not give her the opportunity to answer any questions directed to her. The therapist made it clear that she valued mother's opinion, but stated that she would like to hear from Alicia what she would like to do. Alicia responded by saying she was bored in the house and would like someone of her own age to talk to. She was interested in attending a day centre, but then mother intervened and asserted that the people at the centre were all worse than Alicia and that it would depress her. The therapist agreed that that was a possibility but added that it was worth trying unless mother could suggest another place where Alicia could meet young people. She asked mother if she would take Alicia along to the centre and help her to choose an activity she could benefit from. Mother raised a number of objections and would not commit herself to the plan. The therapist asked her to think it over and said they would discuss it again on her next visit.

2 months

The therapist tried to arrange for the other two children to join them for the next meeting. Nelson made the excuse that he was too busy, but Claire agreed to attend. At the meeting, Claire was openly critical of mother's inability to control Alicia's overeating and said mother was endangering Alicia's health. The therapist intervened to point out that mother was herself incapacitated and needed help with Alicia's care. She asked Claire to suggest one thing she could do to help mother with Alicia. Claire then asked her mother how she could help and Marianne said she should lock up her own food so that Alicia could not get access to it. Claire agreed to this.

The therapist then raised the issue of the day centre. Claire was strongly in favour of this and pressurised Marianne to try it out at least once. She offered to take time off college to accompany them to the centre. After some argument all three agreed to go together and a specific date was fixed.

3 months

The therapist reported that it had proved very difficult to get all the agencies to attend a meeting. Finally a meeting was held with Marianne, the nurse who gives Alicia insulin injections, the psychiatrist responsible for Alicia's care and a member of staff at the day centre. Nobody from the learning difficulties service attended. Discussion focused on control of Alicia's eating problem and her activities at the day centre. It was agreed that the day centre staff would teach Alicia to plan and prepare simple meals within her diet. Marianne was sceptical about her daughter's ability to master even the simplest cooking skills but was prepared to go along with this plan.

Commentary

By being congratulatory, patient and resourceful, the therapist was able to overcome Marianne's antagonism to psychiatric services and personnel. Claire, the healthy daughter, who was direct in her comments to her mother and supportive of the therapist's aims, helped in this task. It is very likely that Marianne has underestimated Alicia's abilities and that she will be able to benefit from the training in food preparation at the day centre. The hope is that giving her more control over the choice of food and its preparation will engender in her a better understanding of the limits of her diet.

The attempt to bring together representatives of all the services required by Alicia was only partially successful. This is a common experience and reflects the lack of coordination of specialised services. Nevertheless the meeting was useful in reaching agreement between the professionals and Marianne on a plan for Alicia, which would be administered by the day centre staff. The opportunity for professionals from a variety of services to meet and discuss a client together establishes a basis for ongoing communication, a necessity for someone like Alicia with both psychiatric and physical problems.

If Alicia settles into the day centre and spends more time away from her mother, it will be necessary to help Marianne to find an activity to fill the gap that opens up in her life. Voluntary work is a possibility, but may be ruled out by Marianne's own physical disabilities. An alternative would be for Marianne to attend a day centre for the elderly, which would enable her to expand her social network.

Family 5. Martin Edwards

History

Martin is aged 39 and has suffered from paranoid schizophrenia since the age of 20. He is the youngest of three children, the older two being from his mother's previous marriage. His biological father died 5 years ago. His mother Jacqueline is aged 70 but is very active. She goes out a lot, plays bridge with a group of friends weekly and travels abroad. Her first marriage ended in divorce and her second marriage in a separation. Martin lived with his father for a while and was very upset by his death. Jacqueline felt that Martin's father turned him against her.

Martin lives alone in a council flat not far from his mother, who does everything for him. She does all his shopping and collects his medication when he asks her. She is so worried about him that she says if she knew she was going to die she would take him with her. On the other hand, when she goes abroad Martin worries about her.

Martin has a girlfriend, Patricia, whom he met when she was on the same psychiatric ward 2 years previously. She is addicted to cocaine and spends most of his money on her habit. She only visits him on his benefits day, which is when she commandeers his money. However, she makes an effort to get him to go out. He is hard of hearing but doesn't use a hearing aid. He gets very paranoid and hears voices, and also misinterprets what he hears from television and people in the street.

This is the main reason why he avoids going out. Patricia is his only friend, although he can get paranoid about her too.

Martin's stepsiblings are Tony, a successful businessman who would like to help Martin, and Susan, who is married with two children.

Presenting problems

How can Martin be persuaded to use a hearing aid? Is it possible to work with his girlfriend, or should she not be involved in the work with him since she has psychiatric problems of her own? What can be done to reduce his mother's overinvolvement?

Formulation

There is an association between deafness and paranoia, so that it is quite likely that Martin's physical disability contributes to his paranoid beliefs that people in the street are talking about him. I once looked after an elderly man who was deaf and suffered from auditory hallucinations. On being asked when he heard the voices, he replied that they only came on at night when he went to bed. I asked him what he did with his hearing aid at night and he told me he turned it off. I advised him to keep it on, and at his next visit he reported that the voices had stopped. Research on sensory deprivation has shown that those without mental illness can develop hallucinations when the input of meaningful information is reduced to a minimum (Leff, 1968). Therefore it would be an important aim to induce Martin to be fitted with a hearing aid and to wear it regularly.

Like many people with schizophrenia, Martin's social network is very sparse. One of the reasons in his case is his paranoia, which is even directed against people he knows well like Patricia. However, given the fact that Patricia undoubtedly exploits him, his paranoid attitude to her has a basis in reality. His mother is extremely overinvolved as shown by the number of things she does for him and her statement that if she died she would want to take him with her, as though he could not survive without her. She would probably benefit from attending a carers' group.

The other people in his network are his two stepsiblings, one of whom, Tony, has expressed willingness to help him. An attempt should certainly be made to recruit him as an ally in the process of improving Martin's quality of life. He is likely to prove easier to work with than either Martin's mother or his girlfriend. His stepsister is another possible ally but may be too busy with her children to offer much. However, her children, Martin's nephew and niece, have the potential to provide him with a valued role as an uncle. People with schizophrenia generally find children less threatening than adults.

Supervisor's suggestions

1. Advise Jacqueline to join a carers' group.
2. Explain to Martin that a hearing aid could help to reduce the frequency with which he hears voices.
3. Invite Tony and Susan to a family meeting with the aim of recruiting Tony to help persuade Martin to use a hearing aid.
4. See Martin together with Patricia and stress the fact that they both have a disability that could be helped. Suggest that Martin encourages Patricia to enter a detoxification programme and that she encourages him to acquire a hearing aid and to use it regularly.

Follow-up

2 months

The therapist encouraged Jacqueline to join a carers' group, which she did and benefited from it. The other group members advised her to withdraw a bit from helping Martin, and she is trying to do this. Martin has been shopping for basic foodstuffs on his own and is generally becoming more active. The therapist is encouraging Patricia to press him to get a hearing aid.

3 months

Martin's siblings attended a family meeting and were very supportive of him. Tony suggested that he could arrange for Martin to have a hearing test and could drive him to the clinic. After some hesitation, Martin agreed to this plan. Susan asked him if he would like to come to her home for tea one weekend, and he accepted.

Commentary

The therapist was faced with the dual difficulty of trying to work with an overinvolved mother and a girlfriend who took advantage of Martin financially in order to fund her substance misuse. In these circumstances it is always worth assessing whether there are healthy siblings available who could be recruited to aid the therapist in his or her task. In this case Martin's stepsiblings were willing to take action to help him and both made useful offers that Martin agreed to take up. In the absence of further follow-up it is not certain that he will keep to his agreement, but at least the meeting achieved the aim of activating part of Martin's very small social network.

The problems of modifying intensely overinvolved relationships when the carer has no other source of emotional satisfaction are formidable. Engagement with a carers' group can be very helpful in a number of ways. The group becomes part of the carer's social network and combats the sense of isolation. It also helps to provide an outlet for distressing emotions and the group members can be much more direct in instructing the carer what to do than the therapist dares to be. Jacqueline has another resource that she appears not to be using, namely her grandchildren. They could provide her with another focus for her need to care, thus taking some of the pressure off Martin. A future aim for the therapist would therefore be to encourage Jacqueline to spend more time with the grandchildren.

It is easy to be very negative about Patricia because of her blatant exploitation of Martin, but she is an important member of Martin's sparse network and needs to be included in the therapeutic work. After all she remains with him even though he can be paranoid about her. Emphasising that they both have a disability puts them on an equal footing. The aim of suggesting that they can help each other overcome their disability is to bring out their capacity for caring and to put a positive connotation on their mutual dependency. There is no information available from further follow-up on the success of this approach.

Family 6. Margaret Brown

History

Margaret is aged 44 and has a mild learning disability. She developed schizophrenia at the age of 19. She struggled at school but can read and write a little. She describes herself as 'a dunce' and reported that she couldn't keep a job, explaining that 'I wasn't very good'. Her sister Janice did well academically, married young and has had four children.

At age 32 Margaret married a man who also had a mild learning disability. There were a lot of difficulties in the marriage, affecting communication and their sex life. After a year they received help from a psychiatric clinic. This continued for a year and then they began to sleep separately. She stopped doing any housework and he started shouting at her. Her parents then took her back into their home, where she has lived for the past 9 years. She has no contact with her husband now.

She has been attending a day centre twice a week and also a yoga class for the general public. At the centre she is in an art group and her paintings are very colourful and bold. The teacher considers them to be of a high standard. She also attends a women's group at the centre and is able to express her feelings. Recently she began missing days and her father went to the centre and reported that she was spending more time at home. Margaret saw the psychiatrist and conveyed her worries about how she would cope when her parents die. They are both in their eighties and have expressed concern about who would care for their daughter after their death.

She was visited at home by a staff member who found that her parents do everything for her. Margaret complained that her life is empty.

Presenting problems

How can Margaret be helped to feel more confident of her abilities and to achieve more independence? She has a good potential to express herself but has no social life outside of the centre and spends all her time with her elderly parents.

Formulation

Margaret's parents have overreacted to her mild learning disability by overprotecting her. As a result, she has very low self-esteem and responds passively to their taking over her activities. Her schizophrenia is well controlled with medication and she has not experienced any psychotic symptoms for some years. Her dependence on her parents naturally generates anxiety about how she will cope without them.

On the other hand, she managed to leave home to get married and kept a difficult relationship with her husband going for several years. During that time she coped with the housework. The break-up of her relationship must have been a severe blow to her confidence and led her into her current position of helplessness. However, her painting reveals a lively and colourful aspect of herself that could be encouraged to emerge more strongly.

There are complex emotional issues between a person with schizophrenia and their healthy siblings. Margaret's sister was successful academically, has a stable marriage and has had four children, achievements that Margaret has failed to attain. She must feel envious of her sister and believe that she is a disappointment to her parents. These feelings may be causing her to distance herself from Janice, who could otherwise be a valuable source of support to her. However, Janice may be anxious that after their parents' death the full responsibility of Margaret's care will fall on her, adding to the task of bringing up four children.

Supervisor's suggestions

1. Explore Margaret's feelings of loss and lack of fulfilment regarding her broken marriage and childless state compared with her sister. Stress her creativity as shown in her paintings.

2.   Congratulate her parents on their care. Allow them to express their anxieties about Margaret's future after their deaths, and discuss how they can help her to develop the necessary self-care skills now.

Follow-up

1 month

The therapist had seen Margaret twice, once with both parents and then with mother only. The parents blossomed on being congratulated on their care of Margaret. At the first visit Margaret was asked what she could do for her parents to thank them for their care of her. She agreed to make them a cup of tea. At the second visit 2 weeks later Margaret offered the therapist a cup of tea. Her mother reported that she had also been doing the vacuuming and washing up. The therapist negotiated that Margaret should make her own bed. The therapist noted that mother looked very sad and asked her about this. She related that her husband goes out to the cinema alone and leaves her to do the housework. The therapist is looking for an art class for Margaret.

Supervisor's suggestions
1.   To see the parents without Margaret and give them the task of going out together and enjoying themselves.
2.   Margaret needs to be engaged in a task while they are out.

2 months

The therapist asked if father would come to the next session. Both women said 'he gets in the way'. She negotiated another task for Margaret – ironing. Margaret then wanted to bake a cake. She bought all the ingredients and successfully made a cake. However, the parents were lukewarm about it. It is evident that they had not really appreciated the effort Margaret had made and that the family members had not yet recognised the importance of giving positive feedback to each other.

Margaret said that father needed a new suit. As a result the parents decided to go on a shopping expedition together. Father said that Margaret would want to come with them but she declined firmly. The therapist negotiated for Margaret to make ham sandwiches for them for their tea in their absence. She reported that the parents often talked about Margaret in the third person in her presence and that they were sometimes critical of her efforts.

Supervisor's suggestions
1.   Concentrate on communication between the family members. Encourage direct communication at all times and reframe criticism as caring.
2.   Assist parents to develop realistic expectations for Margaret.

3.   Link them to the extended family, namely Janice, her husband and their children.

3 months

The shopping trip went very well. Margaret made the ham sandwiches in 10 min and then got bored waiting for her parents' return. She again doubts her abilities.

Mother is very sad that she is alienated from her other daughter, Janice. She is married to an Asian and they are of different religions. The parents are only in touch with one of their grandchildren, a girl who has a daughter of her own.

Father has spent 2 days in hospital because of a heart condition. The parents have made a will and discussed it with Margaret. They have left her the house. At the day centre, Margaret has been talking about death and the possibility of predicting it. She now goes somewhere for organised activities four times a week.

Supervisor's suggestions
1.   Margaret needs more practice of her skills to increase her sense of mastery.
2.   The issue of the parents' mortality is now out in the open and can be discussed.
3.   Negotiate more outings for the parents.
4.   Encourage the family to strengthen the link with the granddaughter.

4 months

Father was in hospital for 10 days to monitor his anticoagulant. Margaret was more active in father's absence but stopped when he returned. He said things like 'She's useless'. On being asked, Margaret said he made her feel that she wasn't there. In his absence Margaret began going to the shop to get the newspaper and has continued with this task. Mother and father continue to go out together and leave Margaret for up to 4 h. The therapist took her to an art class at a local adult education centre as Margaret felt she couldn't manage the journey on her own.

Margaret is overweight and wears unusual clothes – a baseball cap and dresses suitable for an elderly woman. Mother chooses the dresses for her.

The therapist is trying to find a support worker for Margaret. She would like to go to the seaside for the day, as she used to with her parents, but father is unable to travel there and mother won't leave him. Margaret has taken a 3-week break from the day centre.

Supervisor's suggestions
1.   Arrange sessions with Margaret alone in addition to the family sessions. Raise the issues of her diet and clothing. Try to get her to choose from magazines what clothes she likes.

2. Explore the possibility of her attempting to travel by bus.
3. Reframe hostile comments from father and encourage him to thank her for her contributions to the household.
4. Restate the therapist's role and check the family members' current goals.

5 months

Meeting held with the family for review. Father had not attended the previous meeting. Margaret said she felt more confident. She had decided to go on a diet and parents agreed to follow the same diet. Margaret is keen to meet with Janice and her children, and suggested that she write to Angela, her niece. The therapist helped her to write the letter. In fact, she didn't need much help even though mother said she writes rubbish.

Supervisor's suggestion
Meet with the parents on their own for them to express grief and mourning for the loss of their other daughter and their hopes and expectations for Margaret.

9 months

Margaret has moved into a group home. The other residents also have mental health problems but she is the only woman. She has a bedroom of her own but worries about using the bathroom shared with the male residents. No staff are on duty at night. She spends the weekdays in the hostel and weekends with her parents.

In response to her letter, her sister and niece came to visit over the summer and Margaret felt very proud about achieving this rapprochement.

Her antipsychotic medication has been reduced to once per day and she has perked up a lot. Her anxieties about using public transport are partly due to the fact that she gets laughed at because of her odd clothing.

Supervisor's suggestion
The therapist to see the parents on their own to discuss their feelings of loss and to explore ways of filling the gap left by Margaret's move.

10 months

A meeting was held with the parents. They are feeling lost and decided to organise activities for themselves. They were enthusiastic about the therapist's suggestion of going to an Age Concern centre.

Margaret's sister and husband converted to Jehovah's Witnesses, which has deepened the schism in the family.

Margaret has found another bathroom in the hostel that is little used and feels more comfortable with that. She is prompted by her parents to wash and change underwear. She now attends another day centre three times per week and successfully manages two buses to travel there.

The therapist is continuing to meet with Margaret and her parents every 3 weeks.

12 months

Margaret is doing well in the hostel. A support worker is taking her out shopping to buy her own clothes for the first time. She went to the hairdresser for the first time and is painting her nails yellow and orange. She now uses public transport by herself without any problem.

Family meetings now occur monthly. The parents continue to feel emptiness. Father went to the Age Concern day centre but considered it wasn't suitable for him 'or for mother'. However, the therapist asked mother if she would like to go and she said yes.

21 months

The support worker sees Margaret weekly. She goes out with her shopping and to museums. Margaret attends a sewing group and an art group. She had an exhibition of her paintings and drawings but her parents refused to attend.

The hostel staff do everything for her. It is a struggle to get her to do things for herself. The culture in the hostel appears to be that staff do everything for the residents.

Margaret still stays with her parents every weekend. Mother is now almost blind.

Supervisor's suggestions
1. Persuade father to encourage Margaret to wash up after one meal during her visits and to praise her for it.
2. Meet with the hostel staff about encouraging autonomy.
3. Remind Margaret to maintain contact with her niece.

Commentary

These parents had responded to their daughter's learning difficulties and subsequent schizophrenia by abandoning all expectations for her. As a result they made every decision for her and found it impossible to recognise her potential for improvement. Father in particular was very rigid in his attitudes to women, leaving his wife to do the housework while he went to the cinema. Presumably it was his rigidity that created the rift with his married daughter. Sadly the parents failed to visit Margaret's exhibition of her art, passing up the opportunity to admire this demonstration of her success.

Margaret's low self-esteem derived partly from the contrast with her successful sister and partly from the persistent critical attitudes of her parents. Their overinvolvement was gradually reduced by gaining their trust in the first place and then by recruiting them to help Margaret develop self-care skills. This process was made possible by bringing their anxieties about their daughter's care after their deaths into the open. Sometimes the only way to reduce the overinvolvement of older parents is to face them with their mortality. Inexperienced therapists may feel inhibited about talking to parents about their death, but awareness of the problem is inevitably present even when unspoken. The necessary practicalities can only be planned for when the issue is discussed openly, and the therapist may have to take the initiative. Margaret's parents were only able to make their wills and secure Margaret's financial future when their deaths could be spoken about.

The rift in this family between the parents and their older daughter is encountered relatively rarely in this type of work. A therapist may feel that it is outside their remit to tackle this problem but it is bound to have an emotional impact on the person with schizophrenia. In this family the parents concentrated all their emotional needs on Margaret, instead of including Janice, her husband and their children. Healing the rift took some of the emotional pressure off Margaret. In fact, Margaret herself initiated the action that re-established communication with the alienated part of the family.

It is noteworthy that the therapist had never worked with a family previously. It is a tribute to her empathy, warmth and persistence that she was able to help Margaret to leave her parental home and achieve a degree of independence. Unfortunately the staff in the hostel to which she moved were also overprotective, as shown by their performing tasks which the residents should have been encouraged to manage themselves. A number of studies have found critical attitudes towards the residents to be quite common in staff in hostels (e.g. Ball *et al*, 1992). Overinvolvement is rarer but certainly was in evidence in Margaret's hostel. An educational programme for staff, based on schizophrenia family work, has been developed and has been shown to improve their attitudes towards residents and to increase their coping skills (Willetts & Leff, 1997, 2003).

It is fortunate that the therapist was able to work with this family over an extensive period. This is of particular value when family members exhibit overinvolvement, since this set of attitudes takes considerably longer to modify than does criticism.

Family 7. Costas Papageorgiou

History

Costas is aged 43 and lives with his mother Maria. The family emigrated from Cyprus to the UK in the 1970s. The father died 5 years previously. Another brother Regis is married and lives in London. Mother is incapacitated by angina and arthritis in her knees. She cannot get to the shops and relies on Costas to go shopping and run errands.

Costas has a mild learning disability and went to a special school. As a teenager he identified with great singers and dancers and was grandiose. He developed schizophrenia at the age of 20 but was not seen by a doctor. Instead he spent 10 years in his bedroom being cared for by his family. Finally the family sought help from services. He was admitted to a psychiatric hospital with grandiose delusions of identity and spent 5 years as an in-patient. He was then transferred to a day hospital, which he attended for 2 years. Following this he was moved from the parental home to a hostel. However, after a year he moved back with his parents.

Presenting problems

Costas believes he is either very attractive or very ugly and spends a lot of time staring into a mirror. He asks for reassurance and mother reacts by exaggerating his attractiveness. He is socially quite isolated, though he does go to the local shops. Mother does all the cooking.

Costas finds it difficult to accept mother's increasing disability. He gets angry with her and can be quite threatening. His self-care is quite poor and his teeth are decaying. He stays up late to watch television and gets fixated on particular women who appear on programmes.

He is maintained on a depot antipsychotic, received every 2 weeks, plus chlorpromazine at night.

Formulation

Women live longer than men, so it is not uncommon to find a middle-aged person with schizophrenia being cared for by an elderly mother, as in the Papageorgiou family. The mother's life often centres on the care of her sick offspring to the exclusion of all else and the ill person develops an extreme dependency on their mother. Consequently it is very difficult to separate the couple. In this family the dependency was heightened by Costas's learning difficulty and the fact that the family kept his illness hidden for 10 years. Evidence is accumulating that a long duration of untreated psychosis results in organic changes in the brain (Lappin *et al*, 2003), this being one of the arguments for the early detection and treatment of psychosis. Another reason for early intervention is that it prevents carers' emotional responses to the patient from becoming fixed and difficult to modify. Considering the length of time Maria has been caring for Costas, her limited life expectancy and her dependence on her son to shop and run errands, it is unreasonable to consider attempting to separate them at this stage.

Costas's dependence on a caring environment was perpetuated by his spending 5 years in a psychiatric hospital, exposed to all the problems of institutionalisation. It is hardly surprising that he did not manage to remain in the hostel but returned home to his family. Patients cared for by a single elderly relative invariably harbour anxieties about the relative's health and fears of what will happen to them when the relative dies, even if these are unvoiced. Costas deals with these fears by denying his mother's increasing disability and becoming angry about her incapacity, as though it were under her control.

He needs to be helped to express these fears in a direct way and to prepare himself for a future without his mother's care. He should be congratulated on the tasks he does do for her and encouraged to gradually extend them.

However, he is quite handicapped by his persistent delusional concerns with his appearance. These have not responded to his regime of medication and he needs to see a psychologist for exploration of a cognitive approach. This may be hampered by his learning difficulty.

His healthy brother Regis is the only other close family member and might be able to help Costas by taking him out occasionally.

Supervisor's suggestions

1. See Costas individually for an exploration of his fears about mother's ill health and eventual death.
2. Meet with Costas and Maria together to discuss additional ways in which he could help her. It is a useful approach to remind Costas how much his mother has done for him over the years and ask him to think of ways in which he could thank her for her care.
3. Arrange for Costas to see a psychologist for assessment of his suitability for cognitive therapy.
4. Attempt to arrange a family meeting including Regis.

Follow-up

6 months

Costas settled down for a few months after the family was discussed. Then Regis's marriage broke up and he moved back into the family home 2 months ago. Six weeks ago mother phoned to report that Costas was trying to kill Regis because he believed that Regis was maltreating their mother. Costas was punching and kicking Regis's bedroom door. Regis called the police. After they went Costas became angry about their having been called and got more aggressive, so they were called again. More recently Costas hit his mother with a mug. He is becoming more paranoid. He is also worried about having AIDS although he has never had a sexual relationship, but masturbates excessively.

Regis is keen to learn more about schizophrenia and Costas is happy for Regis and mother to know more about his illness. Costas admires Regis's ability to get on with people.

Supervisor's suggestions
1. Educate the family about schizophrenia. Despite the prolonged period Costas spent in hospital, it is possible that Maria was never given education in any form.
2. Meet with the two brothers to discuss their relationship and ways in which Regis could help Costas.
3. See Costas alone about his sexual difficulties. Refer him to a psychologist to work with him on his delusions.

13 months

Since the last discussion he has been admitted to hospital twice. The dose of his depot was increased and since then he has been less aroused. When he settled on the ward he enjoyed being able to talk to people.

A psychologist has engaged well with Costas. They have worked on his belief that he is ugly and that people in the street call him a monster. During therapy there was a re-emergence of paranoid ideas that mother and Regis were conspiring against him.

He has a strong interest in music and sings reasonably well.

Supervisor's suggestions
1. Teach mother and Regis how to defuse tense situations and how to cope with Costas's expression of delusions.
2. Explore the possibility of appointing a befriender with an interest in music. Costas is very isolated but on the ward he proved capable of socialising with the other patients. A befriender with a sympathetic approach might be able to form a good relationship with him and take him to musical events that he would enjoy.

14 months

Maria is very happy to have help with Costas's aggression. Costas agreed that his mother could be seen by the therapist to give her help. There is no progress in finding a befriender. Unfortunately there is a limited supply of volunteer befrienders and they have to be chosen carefully to match a particular individual's needs.

A meeting was held with Costas and Regis. Costas expressed his worry that his brother would take his mother's attention away from him and that they would both try to send him away to a hostel again. Regis was able to reassure him that he was only staying with them until he found a place of his own that he could afford. He also stated that both Maria and he wanted Costas to live at home as long as Maria could care for him. Regis asked Costas if he would like to go with him to a musical evening at a local Greek Cypriot centre. After some hesitation because of the worry that people would stare at him, Costas agreed.

Commentary

It is very unusual these days to find a person with schizophrenia who has been kept at home by their family without treatment for many years. This kind of situation is produced by ignorance of the nature of serious mental illness, pessimism about the possibility of treatment and a strong awareness of stigma. People from minority ethnic groups most often express the latter (Wolff *et al*, 1996). Successful reduction in the period of untreated psychosis has been achieved by early intervention programmes, which include education of general practitioners and the introduction of mental health education classes into secondary schools (Larsen *et al*, 2001).

The people who are most at risk from violence by a person with schizophrenia are family members (Taylor & Gunn, 1999). Yet professionals rarely, if ever, advise them about the warning signs (persistent stare, gritted teeth, clenched fists) or about strategies to defuse tension (time out, carer leaves room, distraction by a task that takes the patient out of the home, e.g. 'Would you please take the dog out for a walk.').

Carers often ask professionals what to do when their relative speaks to voices or expresses delusions. For decades they were given the useless advice to ignore them. Cognitive–behavioural therapy, which has been successful in helping many people with persistent delusions or hallucinations, has not been utilised to advise relatives how to cope with the patient's psychotic symptoms. Maria's attempts to reassure her son when he complains that he is ugly have not benefited him. She needs to be instructed in responses that have been shown to work.

Costas's anger at and suspicion of his younger brother's return home is understandable in view of his lack of success in life compared with Regis. It can be very helpful to hold a joint meeting between the siblings to discuss these emotional issues. In this case Costas's paranoia was defused for the time being and the better feeling between the brothers led to a helpful offer from Regis to take Costas to a musical evening. On Maria's death, Regis will be the only surviving relative of Costas in the UK. If he does not succeed in making any friends by then, he will be reliant on his brother for social contact. Therefore the therapist needs to focus on this relationship, attempting to defuse the negative emotions involved and to resuscitate the warmth that existed before Costas fell ill.

CHAPTER 4

More than one family member with a psychosis

Approximately 10% of people with schizophrenia have a parent with the illness and about the same proportion have an affected sibling. People in the UK of African and African–Caribbean descent have a very high incidence of psychosis, so there is a greater chance of more than one affected member in the same household. In addition, the development of community care, with the consequent freedom of choice of partners, has led to long-standing relationships between two individuals both of whom suffer from a psychotic illness. Each of these partners has to assume a caring role with respect to the other, although sometimes they have an offspring without mental health problems who becomes the carer for both.

When there are two or more affected people in the same household, a very heavy burden falls on the carers. This can be almost intolerable if there is only one person who accepts the caring role. The burden needs to be spread by involving other healthy family members, either within or outside the household. It is also possible to explore with the affected family members ways in which they can adopt some caring activities themselves. This is essential if there are no family members without mental health problems in the household. Individuals then need to see themselves as both patients and carers for each other.

Another issue is the necessity for the carers to appreciate that the experiences and needs of the individual affected relatives are often very different, even when they have the same diagnosis. Their needs are shaped partly by their personalities and partly by the life stage during which the illness appears. The service providers have to resolve the issue of the extent to which the affected members in the same household require different personnel to be responsible for their care. This leads to the problem of balancing respect for confidentiality against ensuring clear and regular communication between the different professionals involved.

Family 8. Derek Baker

History

Derek, aged 33, lives with his parents and is the only offspring. His mother has paranoid schizophrenia and receives an oral antipsychotic from her general practitioner but has not seen him for 18 months. Derek has had schizophrenia and anxiety from the age of 21. Since childhood he has been self-conscious about having a 'funny voice'. He attended university and achieved a 2.2 in English even though he was breaking down at the time. He has never had a steady girlfriend and has sadomasochistic fantasies.

Derek's father has been very abusive towards him, yet at the same time monitors him and manages his medication. Father will not accept that his son is ill – 'He's a bleeding head case'. The therapist has been seeing Derek on a weekly basis for 2 years. He has been to a day centre a couple of times but gets very anxious. He did attend another day centre until it closed. He joined an art class recently but criticised the teacher as being unable to draw.

He has been given education about schizophrenia and has also had anxiety management and speech therapy. His last admission was 18 months ago for a few days.

Presenting problems

Father died of cancer a week ago. Derek has been left with his mother, whom he describes as 'stupid like me'. How can the two be helped to manage together?

Formulation

Derek had a difficult childhood owing to his mother's psychiatric illness and his father's ambivalent attitude. Father accepted a caring role in relation to his son but was overtly hostile and demeaned him. It is likely that this attitude existed before Derek's illness because Derek's self-consciousness about his voice began during his childhood.

He is clearly intelligent and eager to further his education. However, he appears to have adopted his father's critical attitude, as shown by his response to the art teacher. His action in the art class sets himself above the teacher, but he also refers to his mother as 'stupid like me', betraying a deep ambivalence towards himself and his abilities, also reflecting his father's attitude. His sadomasochistic fantasies probably originate from the same source.

Derek and his mother are relatively stable on their medication, but he needs to be admitted to hospital fairly regularly, though for brief periods.

In some respects father's death must be a relief to Derek, but he still needs to mourn his loss, as does mother. It is questionable whether their communication is good enough to help each other with the process of mourning, or whether they each need individual help. They are now both faced with the need to care for the other as well as be cared for. They will have to decide on how to share the tasks involved in running the household.

Supervisor's suggestion

Check the practical arrangements. How will the family manage everyday living? How will they carry on the grief work? There is a need to arrange a meeting with Derek and mother with a therapist for each.

Follow-up

2 months

Derek is becoming more symptomatic but is reluctant to be admitted to hospital. A supportive uncle has helped the two of them. Derek has taken over the cooking of meals from mother. It has been difficult to arrange a joint meeting because the family has always resisted home visits.

Supervisor's suggestions
1. Emphasise to Derek that he has become a carer with new responsibilities.
2. Since home visits are ruled out, try to see Derek and mother together at the team base.

3 months

Derek's mental state continues to deteriorate since father's death. The therapist negotiated with Derek that mother would be invited to a joint meeting by letter. A joint meeting was held at the team base with Derek, his mother and the general practitioner. Mother seems to be managing quite well and is now doing the cooking and washing the clothes. She and Derek go shopping together.

The therapist saw Derek alone afterwards and he talked about his sadomasochistic fantasies.

Supervisor's suggestions
1. The couple have organised themselves to manage the household tasks in a satisfactory way. They appear to have conducted the grief work individually without professional help. Therefore there is little indication for family work now, and each individual should work with their own therapist.

2. Derek is talking openly about his fantasies and might benefit from referral to a sexual disorders clinic.

5 months

Derek deteriorated to the point where he had to be admitted to hospital for 2 weeks. His medication was changed and he is now a lot better.

Supervisor's suggestion
If Derek's self-esteem could be improved it is possible that he would experience fewer relapses. Consider referral to a psychologist for cognitive management of low self-esteem.

6 months

Derek has been discharged from hospital and is now very well. He now wants to keep away from services. He is keen to study English A level, even though he has an English degree.

7 months

He has started two courses, English and computers. He found himself correcting the English teacher and will give up the course. He is enjoying the computer course. He reports that he is getting on better with mother.

8 months

He gave his reason for doing the English course as the opportunity to meet ordinary people.

Supervisor's suggestion
Advise Derek to address his problem of low self-esteem with a psychologist at his local hospital.

9 months

He is doing well and continuing with the computing course.

10 months

He has been non-adherent to medication and is not well again. It is the anniversary of father's death: the timing of this relapse suggests that he has not satisfactorily completed the grief work. He resumed his medication and is now improving. He stopped the computer course because it became too difficult for him. He has made no contact with a psychologist.

Commentary

The father in this family was the carer for both his wife and his son, but was also hostile towards his son, expressing a prejudiced attitude to his mental illness. We do not know whether he reacted similarly to his wife's illness. His death dramatically altered the family dynamics, relieving mother and son of their critical relative but facing them with the need to become carers as well as patients. In the event, they soon learned to share the household tasks equitably and to work cooperatively together.

However, they never received help with mourning and it became clear that Derek was still adversely affected by his father's death, since he experienced an anniversary reaction that led to another hospital admission. In general, mother and son were resistant to offers of professional help, refusing home visits. Derek has a major problem with self-esteem and lack of confidence, shown by his returning to an English A level course despite having a degree in the subject. At the same time he is critical of his teachers, echoing his father's destructive attitude. It is probable that he would benefit from cognitive therapy from a psychologist, but he failed to respond to offers of this service. Also he did not pursue the offer of help with his sexual difficulties.

It is frustrating for a therapist to be faced with clients who have an obvious need for specialist services but who passively or actively resist referral. The optimal response is to keep in contact with the clients, repeat the offers at intervals and hope that in time the pressure of their need will exceed their resistance. Although the initial family meeting that included the general practitioner was sufficient to facilitate a working relationship between Derek and his mother, Derek has considerable potential for personal growth that is likely to lie fallow without individual therapy.

Family 9. Peter Verghese

History

Peter is aged 36. His father comes from Goa and his mother from Paris. He has a sister aged 30 who is married with two young children, and whom he visits regularly. His parents separated when Peter was aged 7 and he has lived with his mother all his life. He had few friends at school, but was a good student and went to university to study accounting. He graduated and obtained a job with an accountancy firm but found that he did not like the work. He is interested in computers and in keeping fit, and has installed exercise equipment in the living room of the flat he shares with his mother. His mother does all the housework, including the cooking. However, he does the shopping. He identifies himself as Goan but has no contact with his father.

He developed schizophrenia at the age of 22 and first came into contact with the services after accusing a stranger of staring at him; he then hit the stranger. He refused to be admitted to hospital and was seen by a forensic psychiatrist who thought the risk of further violence was too slight to justify compulsory admission. He then remained at home untreated for 12 years because his mother would not agree to a section. Eventually the community psychiatric nurse negotiated successfully with mother and Peter was admitted compulsorily 2 years ago. Following some improvement in his condition after treatment in hospital, mother's attitude became more positive.

Peter is now on a novel antipsychotic but is irregular in taking it. He has heard voices in the past but not now. He has a persistent delusion that he is controlled by a computer located somewhere in India. He dresses smartly and goes to clubs to find a girlfriend. However, shortly after beginning a conversation he starts talking about the computer that controls him. He has had a single sexual experience, at university.

Presenting problems

Peter currently attends a Clubhouse where he does a transitional job involving computing. His mother has asked if he could live independently. How can Peter be helped to move out of home? He is very keen to have a girlfriend but sabotages his chances every time by talking about his delusion. Can he be taught to keep it to himself?

Formulation

People whose parents are from widely different cultures can experience difficulty in developing a clear sense of identity. This is particularly so if the parents speak different languages and are not fluent in a common language. Peter's father spoke Tamil with English as a second language and his mother spoke French with English as a second language. Peter lost contact with his father when his parents separated; nevertheless he considers himself to be Goan. His identification with his lost father is likely to reflect difficulties in his self-image, which are inevitably heightened when schizophrenia develops. His belief that the computer that controls him is located in India suggests that he has unresolved feelings that his absent father still exerts an influence over him. If his father can be traced, a meeting with him might help Peter with his problem of identity.

Peter's mother's resistance to his admission to hospital when he first fell ill, and subsequently for a further 12 years, is evidence of over-protectiveness. A further indication of her overinvolvement is her tolerance of having their small living room taken over by his exercise equipment. However, her attitude to his having treatment has changed over the past 2 years, and she is now contemplating Peter moving to his own flat so that she can regain the comfort she has lost.

Peter has a persistent delusion of being controlled, which he shares with relative strangers. People with chronic schizophrenia often have very little to talk about other than illness-related issues, which are likely to bore a new acquaintance or even raise their anxieties. He is obviously intelligent, having a university degree, and looks after his appearance well. However, he will fail to make new friends if he continues to bring up his delusion within a few minutes of beginning a conversation. He is a good candidate for cognitive–behavioural therapy given by a psychologist, who could also coach him in appropriate ways to converse with a new person. He also needs to develop new interests that could furnish him with topics of conversation.

Supervisor's suggestions

1. Find out from mother whether there is a way to contact father.
2. See Peter and mother together to discuss independent living.
3. Refer Peter to a psychologist for cognitive therapy for management of his delusion.

Follow-up

1 month

His delusions are unchanged. He always appears well-dressed and affable. He complained that his mother was depressed and asked the therapist how she could access services.

2.5 months

Peter reported that his mother believes she is being followed. He will be referred to a psychologist for treatment of his persistent delusions, and to a dietician for his weight gain. His mother continues to feel crowded by his exercise equipment and wants him to move to his own flat. She lost contact with her husband many years ago.

He goes to the Clubhouse once a week and has the job of showing people around. His mother is never at home during the day but does everything for him apart from the shopping. However, the therapist judges that he is capable of cooking.

Supervisor's suggestions

1. Meet with mother and Peter and congratulate her on her care of Peter. Tell her she has earned a rest.
2. Peter's anxiety about mother's mental health can be used to motivate him to do one task to relieve her.

4 months

The therapist met with mother and found that she was reinforcing Peter's delusions. He has been referred to a psychologist. He is applying for his own flat and has taken all the documents to the council housing office.

Supervisor's suggestions
1.   Talk to the psychologist about teaching Peter how to approach women.
2.   Find another focus for mother's caring activities.
3.   Educate mother and Peter about schizophrenia and advise her how to deal with his delusions.
4.   Work in collaboration with the occupational therapist. Peter may need help with cooking skills.

5 months

Was reluctant to have home visits to mother's flat but now accepting. He says he won't mind visits to his own flat. He has met the occupational therapist and is happy to have his skills assessed.

9 months

Despite what he said, Peter sabotages visits to their flat. There is a long waiting list for cognitive–behavioural therapy.

Supervisor's suggestion
Offer to meet Peter and mother in the team base.

11 months

Peter is increasingly concerned that mother is ill. She is now talking to herself. He is now prepared to be seen with mother by two therapists.

18 months

Mother is being seen by an old age psychiatrist. She was depressed and paranoid and had become reclusive. The therapist also saw Peter's sister, who will ensure that mother continues her contact with services despite Peter's attempts at sabotage. He won't agree to be seen with mother.

Peter continues to attend the Clubhouse. He is not actively pushing for a new flat. He has applied for a job as a security guard.

Supervisor's suggestions
1.   Discuss the situation with the daughter, now the only member of the immediate family without mental health problems.
2.   In order to tackle mother's social isolation, perhaps she could be encouraged to play more of a role as a grandmother. Suggest seeing mother and daughter together.

21 months

No change in the situation.

Supervisor's suggestion
Attempt to see mother with daughter during mother's visit to out-patients in order to discuss her role as grandmother.

Commentary

Peter was imposing on his mother by dominating her living space with his exercise equipment. She was overinvolved with him, hindering him from developing the skills to live independently. Consequently the initial strategy was to capitalise on her expressed wish for him to move out and to help him learn to look after himself. However, although he appeared to go along with this plan, in effect he sabotaged every attempt to organise meetings to put it into action.

The situation changed dramatically with the appearance of mother's depressive psychosis, about which Peter was exceedingly concerned. As we have noted above, illness in an overinvolved carer is alarming to the dependent patient. The main issue for the future is how far mother will recover from her illness and how much care she herself will need. Her daughter is involved with her own family, including two young children. It is likely that Peter will need to take on a caring role with respect to his mother as she eases out somewhat from her caring for him. A greater reciprocity will therefore need to be achieved between the two of them, as in Family 8.

The aim for Peter to live independently has to be postponed. Meanwhile, efforts need to be made to help him with his persistent delusion. Unfortunately there are currently too few professionals trained in the cognitive–behavioural approach to psychotic symptoms to meet the demand. So Peter will have to wait until he reaches the top of the list. Meanwhile, his mother needs instruction on how to help him with his delusion, instead of reinforcing his belief, but not until she recovers from her own psychotic illness. The loss of contact with his father is unhelpful for Peter, but the therapist can still raise the issue of identification with his father and what being Goan means to him.

Family 10. Melanie Wright

History

Melanie is aged 43 and was brought to England from Jamaica by her parents when she was 6. She trained as a general nurse and worked in hospitals for a few years before developing schizophrenia at the age of 25. She keeps well when taking her depot antipsychotic medication, but often breaks down due to non-adherence. When she relapses she plays music very loud, shouts and reads the Bible a lot. However, she does not belong to a church. She is employed in a general hospital as a nursing assistant and when well she works 12 h a day. She is well liked by the other staff who are tolerant of her relapses. When she is unwell the psychiatric service staff at her hospital look after her.

Her husband Michael is 64, White and is a retired radiographer. He gave up work because he became paranoid about his colleagues. He is obsessional, rigid and deaf. He sees a consultant psychiatrist for his paranoid illness. Melanie complains that Michael doesn't understand her. They have an 8-year-old daughter Rosie. Michael is a good father to Rosie.

In a recent paranoid episode, Michael told the therapist that Melanie was poisoning him and making his urine blood red. He wets the bed. Melanie and Michael have been seen together, but he dominates the conversation and takes up all the time. He complains that Melanie tricked him into getting her pregnant and states that he has been impotent since.

Presenting problems

Recently Michael demanded that the therapist help him obtain more financial benefits for Melanie. When she said it was not possible he became very angry and banned her from the house. How should the therapist deal with his paranoid attitude? Is it possible to work with them together, given his dominating attitude? How can Melanie's adherence to medication be improved?

Formulation

Melanie and Michael are potentially both patients and carers. However, Michael's paranoid attitude to his wife and domination of her makes it difficult for her to fulfil a caring role in relation to him. Recently he has prevented the female therapist from seeing Melanie at home. Her clinical obligation is to Melanie, but Michael also needs a therapist to help him with his paranoid episodes. In this situation it is not possible for a single therapist to work with both partners. Ideally Michael should have a male therapist assigned to him, although there is a possibility of him also becoming the target of Michael's paranoia. The two therapists need to meet with the partners in the team base, since Michael has ruled out home visits. The therapists can of course also see their clients for individual sessions.

On a practical level, Michael needs to be encouraged to acquire and use a hearing aid. Impaired hearing is a contributory factor to paranoid attitudes (see Family 5). It should also improve communication between the partners. The tendency of Michael to dominate any joint conversation with himself and Melanie needs to be addressed. The ground rules for good communication have to be established (Kuipers *et al*, 2002), in particular a fair share for each participant, and active listening promoted.

Rosie has two parents, each of whom has psychotic episodes. Melanie works full-time with long hours and Michael, since his forced retirement, has taken over his daughter's care. He has expressed resentment towards

Melanie for becoming pregnant with Rosie, so that his attitude towards her and the quality of his care need to be assessed. Furthermore, the child's understanding of her parent's mental problems should be explored (see Family 3). Rosie needs to be seen by a child guidance team.

Supervisor's suggestions

1. Michael to be assigned his own therapist.
2. Arrange a meeting at the team base between Melanie and Michael and their respective therapists.
3. Organise for Michael to be fitted with a hearing aid.
4. Arrange that Rosie is assessed by the child guidance team.

Follow-up

3 months

Michael was assigned his own therapist, a man, and welcomed this. A joint meeting was held as suggested. Michael expressed his belief that Melanie and Rosie treat him as an oppressive White male. It emerged that Melanie became very ill after the birth of Rosie. She can care for their daughter physically but does not interact emotionally. She has no family here and no friends. Rosie has been seen by the child guidance team, who consider that she is developing well, without problems.

The male therapist introduced the ground rules for good communication and the issue of a fair share for everyone was used to give Melanie more opportunity to contribute. The matter of a hearing aid for Michael was raised. He was rather reluctant to attend a hearing test, but Melanie pressed him to do so and eventually he agreed.

7 months

A consultant psychiatrist at the hospital where Melanie is employed established a good relationship with her and told her that she would not be allowed back to work unless she took her depot medication. Since then she has been adherent and has needed no more admissions to hospital.

The child guidance team is in touch with Rosie and will monitor her progress regularly. Michael has been fitted with a hearing aid. He attends his out-patient clinic regularly and now has a different general practitioner from Melanie.

Melanie has been discharged from the therapist's case-load.

Commentary

When two partners suffer from a psychotic illness it is advisable for them each to have their own therapist. This is particularly important in this family where the husband has paranoid delusions about his wife. As he also felt that the women were ganging up on him (wife, child and female therapist), it was sensible to choose a male therapist for Michael. He obviously appreciated having a man to relate to.

It emerged that Melanie was very disturbed after Rosie's birth and it is likely that there was a failure of bonding since she has difficulty in relating emotionally to her. It appears that Michael, despite his psychiatric problems, has been a good father to Rosie and her development gives no cause for concern. When a father is mentally ill and cannot work it is common for the mother to become the breadwinner and for the father to take over child care. In this family mother was also ill but better able to function in work than her husband. Despite feeling that the women ('Black') were ganging up on him as a White man, Michael was able to give Rosie good care and make up for Melanie's emotional remoteness. Whether he will be able to cope with Rosie in her teens is a question for the future.

Melanie's poor adherence to medication was dealt with successfully by her consultant psychiatrist, who put pressure on her by threatening to terminate her employment. Thus all the problems raised by Melanie's therapist have been addressed and mostly resolved in a relatively short period of time. Melanie has been discharged from the therapist's case-load, but it is likely that the family will need further input as Michael gets older and Rosie grows up.

Family 11. Pang Family

History

Mrs Pang is aged 65 and was diagnosed as suffering from schizophrenia over 20 years ago. She has four children, the three oldest of whom live with her. Shiu, the oldest, is aged 37 and is the only adult in the household without mental health problems. Li, her sister, is aged 35 and has paranoid schizophrenia and depression. Tsung-Yi, her brother, is aged 33 and has schizophrenia. A healthy brother aged 28 lives in another town. Shiu acts as the carer for her mother and the two affected siblings.

Father divorced mother when Tsung-yi was aged 12. He is now living with a new wife nearby. The only one of his children with whom he is in contact is Tsung-yi.

Li has two daughters aged 4 and 3. She is very labile in mood. She attends classes in English and catering. Mother understands English but cannot speak it. Tsung-yi's English is fluent. He is envious of the attention given to others. The therapist attempted to place Tsung-yi in a hostel. He said he didn't want to move there and ran in front of a bus. The family asserted that they wanted him to continue living with them.

Shiu makes all the decisions and takes family members to all their appointments. She works full time in an office. Li does all the cooking and washing, Shiu does all the shopping and mother does some tidying, but Tsung-yi does nothing.

Presenting problems

Shiu has taken on far too much both as a carer for her whole family and as a full-time worker. How can she be relieved of some of the burden? How can Tsung-yi be persuaded to help with some of the chores? Should efforts be continued to move him to a hostel?

Formulation

The Pangs are a typical extended family such as is found in their native Hong Kong and in other developing countries. Unusually, however, the father has left and three members suffer from schizophrenia. Shiu is the only adult in the home without mental health problems and has taken responsibility for the care of her sick relatives, as well as undertaking a full-time job to bring in some money. This heroic effort demands admiration, but at the same time represents an unacceptable level of self-sacrifice. One-third of carers looking after a single sick relative suffer from depression severe enough to require treatment (Singleton *et al*, 2002), but Shiu's burden is much greater than this. Her sacrifice amounts to overinvolvement and needs to be moderated. Any attempt to persuade her to relinquish some of her responsibilities is bound to conflict with the ethos of a traditional family, with its obligation to care for any sick or disadvantaged relatives. In the Pang family, the imbalance between healthy and sick members must temper this obligation.

The roles of the sick family members need to be assessed, with the aim of determining whether any family member could assume extra responsibilities. Li already does all the washing and cooking and looks after her children. Mother is elderly and is limited in what she can do to help. Tsung-yi is the obvious candidate for extra tasks since he contributes nothing to the family economy at present.

Supervisor's suggestions

1. Given the number of adults in the family, the majority of whom are ill, working with them is too much for a single therapist, and two should be involved. Ideally they should be a woman and a man, so that the latter can form an alliance with Tsung-yi, the only male in the household.
2. Hold a family meeting in which mother's increasing disability is stressed, with a need for others to take over her chores.

3. Explore the possibility of Tsung-yi fulfilling the role of uncle to Li's children. Possibly he could collect them from their nursery school.
4. Ensure that the cultural norms of a traditional extended family are respected with regards both to the duty of care for sick members and the rules governing communication.

Follow-up

2 months

Two therapists, a man and a woman, met with the family, including Tsung-yi. The family was pleased to see them, especially Shiu. Tsung-yi has begun to do some cooking. He is very competitive with Li.

3 months

It has emerged that their father is still involved with the family and is described as very strict. Tsung-yi says that mother is capable of getting to appointments and communicating with professionals.

Supervisor's suggestions
1. Find out mother's care plan from her general practitioner.
2. Reinforce Tsung-yi's responsibility for mother.

8 months

The council have provided a flat for Li, her two daughters and Shiu. After some months they have still not moved in. Shiu is now off sick from work with depression. This followed the break-up of Shiu's relationship with a partner 2 months previously after being together for 5 years. Her partner said he could no longer put up with the amount of time she spent with her family.

Li can cope with her children but Shiu does not believe she is capable. Tsung-yi is improving. He continues to do some cooking. He now says he wants to get a place of his own. Shiu is planning to take Li and the children to mother every evening for a meal after they move.

Supervisor's suggestions
1. Stress to Shiu that she needs to look after her own mental health.
2. Explore her anxieties about what would happen if she allowed Li to take full responsibility for her children. Promote a gradual separation of Shiu from Li.

9 months

The female therapist is focusing on Shiu, who is now establishing boundaries about what she is prepared to do. She is spending a lot of time preparing the new flat. The older of Li's daughters is reluctant to change schools. Shiu is still off work, though her depression is improving.

When the two therapists visit the family, Li makes tea for them and Shiu does all the talking.

Supervisor's suggestions
1. Shiu's domination of the conversation is an aspect of her overinvolvement. The therapists should suggest that mother makes the tea, freeing Li to participate in the discussion.
2. Establish the ground rules for good communication, particularly a fair share for everyone.

10 months

Shiu, Li and the girls have moved into the new flat. After settling in, Shiu returned to work. They all go round to mother's home every evening to eat supper, which is often cooked by Tsung-yi. He has accepted the need to remain in the home to help look after his mother, having received firm instructions to do so by from father.

Commentary

In Western societies the therapist's aim for a young person with schizophrenia is to achieve independence from their family of origin. This is not appropriate when working with a traditional extended family. Even when a son or daughter leaves the family's residence, they remain closely attached to the whole family. This enduring attachment plus the strong sense of obligation to care for sick relatives means that the usual Western standards of rating overinvolvement have to be modified.

The Pang family is particularly unfortunate in having three members develop schizophrenia, a situation exacerbated by the absence of the father from the household. It naturally fell to Shiu, the only adult in the home without mental health problems, to take on a caring role for the whole family. However, she went beyond her culture's normative expectations in also working full-time, and in her attitude to her sister Li, whom she considered incapable of being a good mother to her daughters, despite evidence to the contrary.

The consequence of her overinvolvement was the break-up of her long-standing relationship with a boyfriend and the development of depression, which was so severe that she took sick leave from her job.

The two therapists were able to work effectively with the Pangs, partly through respecting their cultural traditions. Eventually part of the family was enabled to separate and form a smaller unit, but still in close daily contact with the other relatives. The male therapist formed a good relationship with Tsung-yi, who progressively became more active in the household. Initially it appeared that their father was remote from the family but later it became clear that he still wielded considerable influence. At a crucial point in the therapists' work with the family, he stepped in to ensure that Tsung-yi remained as mother's carer. His continued relationship with his son probably reflects the special place of males in traditional families.

Family 12. Donald and Eric Bright

History

Donald is aged 44 and Eric is 26, the youngest of five children who keep in regular contact with each other. The two brothers live with their elderly father who has diabetes and Parkinson's disease. Their mother died 7 years ago. Both brothers have schizophrenia. Eric's first contact with the services was at age 18. He has been admitted several times with paranoid delusions, hallucinations, aggression towards objects and suicidal ideas. He is maintained on a depot antipsychotic and currently has few positive symptoms but considerable negative symptoms. He will attend an out-patient clinic and appointments with a community psychiatric nurse but refuses to go to a day centre.

He is a sociable person, easy to get along with, has a willingness to discuss his problems openly and has some insight. His intelligence is below average but not at the level of learning disability. He is able to function independently but is easily led and often requests his father to speak or act for him.

Donald has been ill since the age of 22. He has been stable on medication for many years and mainly exhibits negative symptoms. He is less outgoing than his brother and also less active. The three men are heavily dependent on one another and spend the majority of their time together at home. Brothers and sisters live locally and come round to visit, bringing the grandchildren, but do not invite Eric and Donald to their homes.

Presenting problems

The three men express concern at what will happen when the father dies. How can father be persuaded to give his two sons more autonomy?

Formulation

It is unusual to find a solitary father acting as carer for his children, since women live longer than men. Mr Bright has been a joint carer for nearly 20 years and the sole carer for both sons for the past 7 years since, his wife died. He is physically ill and moderately incapacitated by Parkinson's disease, so that he rarely goes out. His life is centred on the care of his sons and he has no other interests apart from watching television. He is visited by the other children and the grandchildren occasionally, but is not deeply engaged with them. His life would have little purpose without his caring role, which occupies his time and provides him with job satisfaction. For these reasons, it is very difficult for a therapist to persuade him to give up some of his responsibility for the sons. The only lever to effect change is his mortality (see Family 6), of which all three men are aware.

The healthy siblings make little effort to socialise with Eric and Donald. This could be because of their anxiety that they may be expected to take over their care after father's death. There may also be an irrational fear of Eric or Donald harming their children. A meeting with them could reduce these anxieties.

Supervisor's suggestions

1.   Congratulate father on his care of his sons. Point out that his physical ill-health must make it difficult for him to carry out all the chores he tackles. Suggest that each son undertakes to help him with one of the household tasks.
2.   With the family's agreement, make contact with the healthy siblings with a view to them inviting Eric and Donald to visit.

Follow-up

1 month

The therapist visited the three men in their home. At the team base they tend to avoid the main issues, but the meeting at home was much more focused. They talked about feeling let down by the rest of the family. The therapist concentrated on their strengths. Father does everything for them and is too anxious to spend a night away from them. The therapist suggested a division of household tasks.

4 months

Father was admitted to hospital with a chest infection and with his diabetes out of control. The two sons took over the running of the household and managed quite well.

6 months

Father is now back home. The situation returned to what it was before he was admitted. Donald continues to do very little. Father is cooking all meals and looking after his sons. The therapist saw Eric about attending a computer course. He made one visit to a local day centre.

Supervisor's suggestions
1.   Explore the anxieties of each member about father's future health.
2.   Reassure father that his role as carer is not going to be taken away from him.

7 months

Eric's therapist saw all three men together. Father was unhappy because Eric missed his depot injection. The therapist asked about the financial arrangements. Eric pays for the electricity, telephone and television licence. Father gets £60 per week from each son and uses it to pay for cigarettes and for household expenses. He does the laundry.

Donald has become a bit more active: he takes the dog for a walk twice a day. He also vacuums and tidies up.

Father asked to visit the day centre which Eric attends.

Supervisor's suggestions
1. Hold another family meeting to explore anxieties about the future for all of them.
2. Suggest that father teaches each son one simple thing.

8 months

A family meeting was held. Eric's medication has been reduced and he is now getting more psychotic. He takes a taxi to the emergency clinic to talk to someone. Donald's medication is also being reduced gradually as it is above the recommended limit.

The therapist persuaded the sons to cook breakfast under father's supervision. It was agreed that the sons would take it in turn to do the cooking and shopping.

They are planning to go to Portugal together for a holiday. Donald is reluctant to go.

9 months

Donald was admitted to hospital after an attack of anxiety and collapse. Nothing was found to be wrong with his physical health. His anxiety made him drink a lot of water. This anxiety was about father dying, but he could not talk to him about it. As a result of his admission one of their sisters, Susan, offered to look after Eric and Donald when father dies. Father was very pleased with this arrangement.

Father sabotaged the cooking rota that had been agreed. Donald is feeling very confused because father took over his cooking day.

Eric's medication has been changed to a novel antipsychotic and he has become very active. He is now decorating their home. Donald has a standing arrangement to attend a local day centre three times per week.

Supervisor's suggestion
The therapist needs to re-emphasise to father that his role is supervisory.

10 months

Since reducing his medication Donald has been better: not so tearful and less confused. He attends the day centre one to three times per week.

Donald wants a girlfriend but has difficulty socialising. He won't go to parties held by his relatives and he won't engage with services apart from the day centre, and won't eat there.

Supervisor's suggestion
Consider finding a befriender for Donald.

13 months

Eric expressed a wish to move to a flat next door to Susan, who agreed to help look after the brothers when father dies.

15 months

Susan now says that her family comes first and so the plan has collapsed. The sons are now sceptical about her actually helping when the time comes.

Supervisor's suggestions
1. Therapist to tell the family that she is thinking of stopping family sessions as they do not want to change. Say that they are comfortable with the status quo and that father will live a lot longer.
2. From now on therapist to see only Donald as his keyworker.

19 months

Susan now only visits them when she is called by father. Donald attends the day centre but only sits in the current affairs group without saying anything. The therapist sees him twice a week and encourages him to talk about himself. She is trying to improve his self-image. The dosage of his medication continues to be reduced.

22 months

Donald's medication is now at the recommended dosage but his antidepressant has been increased. The therapist thinks he is much better. Eric continues to decorate the flat with help from father. Father is still doing all the cooking and shopping.

Supervisor's suggestion
The therapist should liase with the supervisor at the day centre to approach Donald about preparing meals there.

27 months

The three men went on a caravan holiday together by the sea for a week. Eric stopped his medication just before the holiday. He went out to a pub and felt a sense of freedom, and generally enjoyed himself. He resumed his medication on returning home. He has become more outgoing and is shopping by himself in supermarkets.

Supervisor's suggestions
1. Eric's therapist to liase with Donald's therapist about reducing father's overinvolvement.
2. Encourage Eric to do more shopping.

28 months

Father gets frustrated with Donald, who is very negative. Eric is talking about getting a job. He would like to be a courier, as he has a motor bike. Donald has agreed to a joint meeting with the two therapists.

Supervisors suggestion
Eric might benefit from an aptitude assessment to help him choose an appropriate job.

30 months

Eric's idea of being a courier fizzled out. He is now thinking of shelf-stacking in a supermarket. Eric could go to a job-training centre for an occupational assessment. There are no available befrienders for Donald at the moment. The three men have been invited for Christmas dinner by Susan.

Supervisor's suggestion
Hold a family meeting to discuss their anxieties about social occasions.

Commentary

The therapist's aim of encouraging the brothers to become more active and to do more for themselves was hindered by Donald being over-medicated: the dosage was well above the recommended maximum. A gradual reduction in the dosage to below the maximum resulted in an improvement in his mood and activity. However, the father was unable to move to a supervisory role and sabotaged attempts to reduce the amount he was doing for his sons. Attempts were made to calm his fears that he was being displaced from his caring role but did not produce the required shift.

In view of the obdurate nature of this family problem, I suggested a paradoxical intervention (Selvini Palazzoli *et al*, 1978), a strategy I rarely use because to me it smacks of manipulation. I advised the therapist to tell the family that further meetings together were unnecessary because the three men were comfortable the way they were and father still had years of life ahead of him. The therapist then discontinued family meetings and returned to her original role of seeing only Donald. Following this, Eric became more independent and even considered taking a job, although this cannot confidently be ascribed to the paradoxical intervention.

Since father found it impossible to allow Donald to do some of the cooking at home, an alternative strategy was suggested of organising this activity for him at the day centre he attended. There was no follow-up on this approach.

Father's admission to hospital prompted his daughter Susan to promise to look after her brothers when he died. Unfortunately she withdrew this offer on reflection, feeling that her commitments to her own family took priority. This obviously must be the case but in the future she should be encouraged by the therapist to take a more active role in helping the brothers to socialise, particularly as she was willing to have them join her family for Christmas. She would need to be reassured that there would be a limit to the demands on her time, as her brothers are much more capable of looking after themselves than appears at present. Faced with the failure to alter father's attitude and behaviour, a therapist needs to explore other solutions to the problem, such as the paradoxical intervention used in this family with some success.

Family 13. Hassan Qureshi

History

Hassan and his identical twin brother Kassim are aged 28. Both came to the UK from Pakistan to study. They work in a cousin's restaurant and live in a room above the restaurant where they share a double bed. Hassan went back to Pakistan for an arranged marriage 2 years ago. The marriage was never consummated and he is now divorced.

Hassan became suspicious of customers in the restaurant. He saw some of them turn into dogs in the street and read the Koran to them. Kassim took him to an emergency clinic, where Hassan tried to strangle him and was admitted to a psychiatric ward. On examination he admitted to hearing voices since the age of 15. They tell him he is homosexual and will never get another woman. The voices also tell him he is stupid for not setting up a business here. He and Kassim plan to set up a restaurant together. He was given a diagnosis of schizophrenia and started on medication. An older brother in Pakistan also has schizophrenia.

Hassan's English is not good and Kassim translates for him. He does everything for his twin. Kassim is depressed and has been seeing a psychiatrist in the service for 3 months. He has been attending a carers' group and has had his own community psychiatric nurse for 8 months.

Hassan was prescribed a novel antipsychotic but complained of side-effects and refused to take it. He was seen with an interpreter and agreed to take a monthly depot injection. He seems more outgoing now.

Presenting problems

How can Kassim be disengaged from his brother's care to allow Hassan to become independent of his twin?

Formulation

When one identical twin has schizophrenia, the other twin will develop the illness in around half the cases. Kassim does not have schizophrenia but he has depression severe enough to require psychiatric treatment. This could be independent of his brother's illness or could be a result of the strain of caring for Hassan. His depression can be used as a lever for change, as it can be pointed out to him that he needs to spend some time and energy caring for himself.

The twins share the same bed and Kassim does everything for Hassan, evidence for considerable overinvolvement. The difficulty of separating the twins is compounded by the fact that Hassan relies on Kassim to be his translator. One important intervention would be to ensure that Hassan has lessons to improve his English.

Hassan has a problem with his sexual orientation. He failed to consummate his marriage and his voices tell him he is homosexual. Possibly his extremely close relationship with his twin, both emotionally and physically, has influenced his sexual orientation.

Supervisor's suggestions

1. Convene a joint meeting between the two brothers and their two community psychiatric nurses.
2. Explore their worst fears about separating. Give Kassim permission to give up some responsibility for Hassan.
3. Arrange English lessons for Hassan.

Follow-up

2 months

The twins' mother died of heart disease in Pakistan. Hassan went to be with her while she was dying. He came back extremely well. He met a girl while in Pakistan and is excited about her. He is going back to Pakistan for a ceremony. The brothers have inherited two flats in Pakistan that they are considering selling to provide capital to start a takeaway food shop. They have now stopped working in the cousin's restaurant. Kassim's therapist is helping him with mourning for his mother.

4 months

While Hassan was in Pakistan, his therapist met with Kassim. He expressed concerns about Hassan picking up prostitutes. He is having second thoughts about living with Hassan when they move from their current accommodation above the restaurant. Kassim reports that he is keeping the books for his cousin who runs the restaurant.

Two weeks ago the therapist held a joint session with the brothers. Hassan had difficulty concentrating so Kassim acted as his translator. Kassim reported that when Hassan runs out of clean clothes he wears Kassim's. The therapist set Hassan the task of going to the laundry with Kassim, who would organise the wash. Hassan did not succeed in doing this. The therapist encouraged Kassim to tell Hassan that he could not do everything for him any more. Hassan responded by saying he would find a wife.

Supervisor's suggestions

I suspected that there was some confusion between the therapists over the limits of their roles and made a check on the number of professionals involved with the two brothers. Kassim and Hassan each see a different psychiatrist and community psychiatric nurse. An additional two community psychiatric nurses see the brothers together. Kassim recently contacted a carers' organisation and asked for a social worker to be involved. If his request were to be granted, there would be seven different psychiatric professionals involved with the two brothers. This is a reflection both of Kassim's overinvolvement and of the lack of clear boundaries between the twins. Kassim's overprotective behaviour is probably motivated by survivor guilt: the fact that his identical twin developed schizophrenia but he escaped.

1. Hassan's therapist was advised to call a meeting of all the professionals involved in order to rationalise care.
2. Kassim's therapist needs to explore his sense of guilt concerning his twin's illness.

13 months

Kassim no longer attends a psychiatrist as his depression has receded. He was seen by his community psychiatric nurse for a short period of group work to help him deal with mother's death. Another community psychiatric nurse gives Hassan his depot medication. He has moved to a flat of his own which Kassim shares. They now sleep in separate bedrooms. Two other therapists are still seeing the brothers together. Kassim is looking for a suitable property to open a café. Their family want them to return to Pakistan but they feel there are few business opportunities there. Kassim attends college to learn catering and works in a café in the evenings.

Hassan put on a great deal of weight as a result of his medication and reached 18 stone. He is keen to lose weight and managed to reduce by 2½ stone over 3 months. The brothers go swimming together. Hassan phones Kassim several times an evening to report on his weight. He eats in Indian restaurants during the day.

Supervisor's suggestions
Hassan to keep a weight chart and report back to Kassim at the end of each day.

Commentary

Overinvolvement is relatively uncommon in siblings, but in this family it developed in the unaffected identical twin of an individual with schizophrenia. Survivor guilt is quite usual among the mentally healthy siblings of a person with a psychotic illness, but is inevitably more intense when the individual who escapes the illness shares the same genome with the affected family member. Kassim's overprotectiveness was heightened by Hassan's inadequate command of English, but he probably failed to take the necessary steps to improve his fluency because he wished to perpetuate his dependent status. This is supported by his statement that if Kassim is to curtail some of his caring activities, he, Hassan, will need to find a wife.

It became apparent from the reports of Hassan's therapist that there were a surprising number of psychiatric professionals involved with the twins (six) and that there was some confusion as to who was supposed to be doing what. This is an example of the way in which an overinvolved carer can transmit their sense of guilt to a whole team, who then fall over themselves trying to do too much for the carer and the patient. There was an added complication in this family, namely the lack of a clear boundary between the two brothers (they shared the same bed), which was also reflected in the muddle over roles in the team.

The optimal way to rationalise the professional care given to such a family is to hold a meeting of all the professionals involved and decide on the *minimum* input required. In this case the recommended meeting did not take place. However, when Kassim recovered from his depression, following grief work with his therapist, his psychiatrist bowed out and other professionals gradually withdrew.

The twin's mother's death catalysed a change in both twins. Hassan made the journey to his homeland by himself, met a girl he became excited about, and returned to the UK in a much better state. Kassim's grief work for his mother had wider effects in relieving his depression, which pre-existed the bereavement, and in freeing him to some extent from his sense of responsibility for his twin. He became able to consider living apart from Hassan. Some practical progress was made in that they moved to a new flat and occupied separate bedrooms. Futhermore, Kassim started attending college during the day and took on an evening job in a café, thus spending much less time with Hassan.

Hassan remains quite dependent on Kassim, as shown by his frequent reporting on his weight to his brother every evening. I suggested that he keep a weight chart and report to Kassim once at the end of the day to wean him off this constant phone contact.

In conclusion, the twins have begun to establish separate identities and daily activities, but further work needs to be done on boosting Hassan's confidence and reducing Kassim's overprotectiveness.

CHAPTER 5

Parents in a conflictual relationship or separated

Lidz and his colleagues in the USA studied 17 families consisting of two parents and an adult offspring suffering from schizophrenia. Their team conducted repeated interviews with each family from a psychoanalytic perspective. From their observations of family interactions they formulated two kinds of parental dysfunctional relationships: 'marital schism' and 'marital skew' (Lidz *et al*, 1957). Marital schism refers to a conflictual relationship between the parents manifested as a failure to cooperate; marital skew refers to a situation in which one parent is dominant and the other passive, thus avoiding open conflict. This group of researchers noted that marital schism predominated in families where the patient was male and in which the mother was dominant and the father passive. They postulated that these parental constellations were the cause of schizophrenia.

Their conclusions were faulty for a number of reasons: they studied a very small sample of highly selected families, they had no comparison samples of families caring for patients with other psychiatric illnesses, or samples of families with offspring without mental illness, and they failed to consider the possibility that the disturbed parental relationships were a response to the development of schizophrenia in an offspring. Their theory deserves little credence nowadays when one considers that one in three marriages in the UK now ends in divorce, and other partners live virtually separate lives although in the same household. Disturbed relationships between partners are so common that they could not possibly be the cause of a relatively rare condition such as schizophrenia. However, parental conflict can readily generate stress for offspring with a psychotic illness, resulting in an exacerbation of the symptoms. Each parent may try to recruit both healthy and ill offspring to their camp, producing a conflict of loyalty. Once the parents have separated, patients may shuttle between them, creating an additional instability in their lives.

The daily problems posed by caring for a person with a psychotic illness are often very difficult to solve. Solutions simply cannot be worked out when the parents are in conflict or not even on speaking terms. A common source of conflict is a difference in opinion as to how to treat the patient. The mother may complain that the father is too hard on the patient and he asserts that she is too soft. Healthy siblings may take on a caring role in the absence of parental cooperation and become very burdened.

Therapists are faced with the problem of engaging both parents and attempting to improve their cooperation in the patient's care without becoming drawn into the marital conflict. It is important to make a clear distinction to the parents between their interpersonal problems and the difficulties posed by the care of the patient. At some stage the therapists may consider offering the parents a referral for couple therapy.

Family 14. Polly Farmer

History

Polly is aged 23 and is in her third year at university, studying history and philosophy. She started to feel her lecturer was referring to her and became perplexed and questioning. She was referred to a psychiatric clinic and was started on antipsychotic medication. Her older brother Mike has accompanied her to each appointment, having given up his job.

She responded well to the medication but stopped taking it and went back to university. She relapsed quickly and was wandering around saying people had glazed eyes, and was hearing voices commanding her to cut her wrists and lie in the bath.

At first her parents would not get involved, so that Mike took on the role of carer. Mike is living in his own flat but has daily contact with the family through the phone or visiting. The parents eventually admitted that Polly had had difficulties for some years in the form of an eating disorder with self-induced vomiting up to six times a day. There was no history of bingeing. Her weight increased on the antipsychotic.

Father is self-employed as an insurance salesman and has an alcohol problem. Mother is a housewife and keen gardener. Polly reported that she has had a poor relationship with mother since her childhood and finds her a cold person.

Polly's sister Sophie is a year older and has just finished her degree, getting a high grade. Polly is pleased for her sister but envious of her success.

A family meeting was held with the parents and the three children. Father was quiet and pleasant but did not say much. He was caring towards Polly and warmer than mother. Mother was more active than father. She was not critical of Polly but showed little warmth towards her. Mike was the most active, tending to speak for Polly, whereas Sophie was very quiet. Neither in this session nor in a subsequent one did mother and father sit together or address any remarks to each other.

Polly did not respond to the resumption of the antipsychotic, so it was changed to another drug.

Presenting problems

Polly currently has prominent negative symptoms but gets up with prompting from mother. She has made a firm decision to return to university. She lived away from home during term times. Can the parents be encouraged to take more of a caring role and relieve Mike of the responsibility he has taken for his sister? Should Polly try to return to her studies at this stage?

Formulation

Mr and Mrs Farmer are evidently in a state of what has been called emotional divorce. They do not communicate with each other in family meetings or show any physical closeness. Their failure to take action concerning Polly's eating disorder, which began several years ago, and their initial reluctance to help with her current problem indicates that they are paralysed by their inability to form a working alliance.

Her brother Mike stepped into the gap to help Polly but unfortunately shows signs of overinvolvement: he attended all her appointments with her and speaks for her in meetings. Her sister Sophie appears uninvolved, but this may be her response to the parents' discord and Mike taking over.

The therapist has to tread a fine line between attempting to resolve the conflict between the parents to enable them to help Polly and becoming involved in marital therapy. She has to bear in mind that her client is Polly, not the family. If she considers that marital therapy is needed and might be acceptable to the couple, she should present them with the option of being referred to a clinic for therapy or engaging with her for this purpose.

Polly's eating disorder preceded the schizophrenia by several years and is likely to be related to the dysfunctional parental relationship. She needs referral to a dedicated eating disorders service, since the problem will not disappear as a result of treatment of the schizophrenia. For people with an eating disorder still living with their parents, the most effective treatment is family therapy (LeGrange *et al*, 1992). However, there is likely to be difficulty in persuading her parents to agree to this.

Polly's intention to return to university presents a common dilemma. Patients recovering from a first episode of schizophrenia are understandably concerned to resume their life as soon as possible. However, returning to a demanding educational course too soon inevitably leads to failure and further damage to their confidence and self-image. It is necessary to advise patients and their family that there is often a prolonged convalescent period before the person is ready to resume a course of study. It is particularly difficult for Polly to accept a delay because she is in her final year at university and envies her older sister's academic success.

Supervisor's suggestions

1. It is advisable to have two therapists working with this family owing to the number of members (five) and the schism between the parents. A male therapist should work together with the female community psychiatric nurse. See the family every 2 weeks instead of monthly as at present, and give them an education programme.
2. Meet with the parents on their own to determine whether it is possible for them to cooperate in caring for Polly.
3. In order to ease Mike out of his caring role, find out why he has given up his job.

Follow-up

2 weeks

The first session of education has been given. Father was absent due to illness. Polly was shocked by the diagnosis and Mike was in tears. Mother responded best, recognising that Polly had been ill for years. It emerged that mother and father do not share a bedroom and do not eat together.

Polly has now been prescribed a novel antipsychotic, but is still getting ideas of reference from the television.

Supervisor's suggestions
1. Continue meeting with the whole family, including father, to give further education.
2. Mike's tearful response to Polly's diagnosis is confirmation of his overinvolvement. See Mike and Polly together and encourage them to talk about the split between the parents.

2 months

Sophie has gone to India to take up a job and Polly wants to visit her there. She has begun reading novels again. She was seen on her own by the male therapist in the absence of her community psychiatric nurse and revealed that she believed an ex-boss of hers is behind her delusional experiences. She is convinced that he is trying to control her.

Father attended the last education session and Polly sat between mother and father. She reported that before her illness she felt closer to father but now feels closer to mother.

Supervisor's suggestion

Polly's sitting between her parents indicates that she is either protecting them from angry interchanges or that she believes she is responsible for holding them together, or both. Get mother and father to sit together, using the argument that this might improve communication in the family. Ask them to talk to each other about something non-threatening, like a book they have both read, or, if possible, about their relationship and the impact of Polly's illness.

3 months

The therapists were able to persuade mother and father to sit together. Father talked about his old job in the city. Mother was disinterested and interrupted to ask about a new drug for schizophrenia. Polly sat between the two therapists. Mike was absent. The therapists encouraged Polly to share her psychotic experiences with father and mother. She said she thought she was being spied on by her old boss and by Mike's ex-partner Paul (this was the first time it emerged that Mike was gay). She said that programmes on television commented on her own family and that she thought her parents also believed this. They denied it.

She is now going out for walks with mother and enjoying it. She is also being seen individually on a weekly basis by her community psychiatric nurse.

Supervisor's suggestion

The meetings with her community psychiatric nurse provide an opportunity to discuss her lack of a boyfriend. Explore her attitude to men and to her body, as eating disorders usually involve a disturbance of body image and attitudes to sex.

4 months

Mother and father sat together and Polly was between the two therapists. Her medication has been changed to a conventional antipsychotic and she is much better, smiling and laughing in the session for the first time. She went to an art exhibition with mother. She is still keen to travel to India in 2 months' time and was given the task of reading a book on India. She has started attending a typing class. She has written to Sophie telling her the diagnosis. She no longer talks about her delusions.

Mike has obtained a post as a manager of a computer shop and is less involved with Polly.

Supervisor's suggestion

See whether Polly wants her friends informed about how to cope with her symptoms.

5 months

Polly is feeling better and challenging things more, but her psychotic symptoms are quite resistant to medication. She has recently become depressed and cut her wrists a week ago. She did not want anyone to know, but Mike discovered it and reported it. Her vomiting has increased and she leaves the vomit on the toilet seat without making any attempt to clean it up. She has delusions of reference relating to her being fat. She is drinking more alcohol: a bottle of wine and half a bottle of Baileys in an evening. Mother now retires upstairs in the evening to watch television. Polly would not drink in front of mother.

Supervisor's suggestions
1. Discuss Polly's drug-resistant delusions with a cognitive psychologist.
2. Refer Polly to an eating disorders clinic.
3. Teach the family how to calculate alcohol units and see the parents together to discuss ways in which they can help her restrict her alcohol intake.

6 months

The community psychiatric nurse offered mother a session together with father. She phoned back and refused. Mike has dropped out of sessions because of his new job.

The therapist raised the issue of Polly's drinking with her father and explained that he was a poor role model for her. Polly has stopped drinking now. Father reported that Polly has been vomiting since her teenage years. She has now been referred to an eating disorders clinic. She has also been inducted into a cognitive remediation project and attends four times a week. Mother reports that it is easier to get her out of bed.

Mike sent the therapists a fax asking them to deal with more general family issues.

Supervisor's suggestions
1. Mother's refusal to be seen together with father in order to help with Polly's problems indicates a deep rift between the parents. Consequently it would endanger the work with Polly for the therapists to suggest that they might tackle the relationship between the parents, as Mike is requesting. Reply by letter to Mike with copies to each family member stating that the therapists respect the lifestyles that mother and father have established and have no intention of changing them. The remit is to help the family to cope better with Polly's behaviour due to the illness.
2. The way Polly leaves her vomit on the toilet seat for all to see has been her way of communicating her distress in the absence of any

69

possibility of talking about it to her parents. Hopefully she will be helped to voice her emotional concerns to the eating disorders specialist.

7 months

Polly took a serious overdose of 70 paracetamol and regretted it 2 h later and induced vomiting. Next day she was vomiting and drowsy. She saw her community psychiatric nurse 3 days later. She was admitted to a local psychiatric unit. She had started superficial cutting of her arms before the overdose.

8 months

Two family meetings were held on the psychiatric ward with father, Mike and Polly. Mother refused to come. The next session will include Sophie, who is back from India on leave.

Polly's medication was changed to clozapine and she was discharged.

Supervisor's suggestion
In view of the impossibility of having mother and father attend the same meeting, suggest that they alternate at meetings.

10 months

Two more family sessions were held on the ward including Sophie. She was upset that she had not been told about the overdose. The two sisters were mutually supportive in the sessions. Father just went to sleep.

Polly has had a partial response to clozapine: the voices are more distant and she is better able to sleep. She has finished the cognitive remediation project and has started reading again. She has been offered attendance at a drop-in centre but has not yet been. She has a few friends from university and maintains tenuous contact with them.

Mike sent a message cancelling the family meetings.

Supervisor's suggestion
Send a letter to the family stating that the therapists respect their decision not to continue but saying they are open to future contact.

11 months

Polly's dose of clozapine has been increased and has now reached 300 mg/day. However, hypotension is a problem. A care programme review meeting was held recently with Polly, Mike and father. She is improving: the voices are now so indistinct that she cannot hear what they are saying. She has started to attend a Clubhouse and is also doing voluntary work with Mike. She travels with him on a minibus on its rounds to bring elderly people to and from an Age Concern centre. She initiated a visit to the cinema with father and Mike. However, she still feels she is being monitored.

Supervisor's suggestion

Mike seems to have established a healthier relationship with Polly and is helping her recovery. The therapists should see Polly and Mike together to explore other ways in which he could help her.

12 months

Polly refused to have a meeting with the therapists and Mike.

24 months

Polly is doing well. She works in a clerical job 1½ days per week. Clozapine has helped a lot and her psychotic symptoms are very well controlled. Her community psychiatric nurse is seeing her every 3 weeks. Sophie has returned from India and is living at home again.

Commentary

The emotional divorce of the parents over many years has had a significant effect on their three children. Sophie took a job in India to escape from the atmosphere in the home, Mike chose a homosexual partner and Polly developed an eating disorder in her teens. Despite the clear evidence of Polly's disturbance, her parents did not seek help from the services. The attitude of not wanting to deal with problems pervaded the whole family, with the exception of Mike, who welcomed the therapists' intervention and wanted them to tackle issues beyond Polly's psychiatric symptoms. Although they were able to keep both mother and father together in a few sessions, this did not last and mother made it absolutely clear that she would not join father in a meeting. When father did attend a session with Polly in the hospital, he fell asleep – a way of absenting himself.

Despite these immense difficulties, the therapists managed to remain engaged with Polly, Mike and Sophie by sending letters to all the family members stating that their work was limited to helping Polly recover. Even so, at different stages Mike sent a message cancelling family meetings and Polly refused to be seen together with Mike.

Undoubtedly Polly's recovery from schizophrenia was greatly aided by clozapine, but other contributions came from psychological treatment of her cognitive problems, specialist referral for her eating disorder and the interventions of the therapists. They succeeded in halting her incipient alcoholism by changing father's drinking patterns, and reduced Mike's overinvolvement, enabling him to find a job and then to play a therapeutic role in her rehabilitation. Polly's return to her studies was postponed and she successfully undertook part-time work in open employment. She now has the potential of additional support from her sister, and with both her siblings taking on a caring role she stands a chance of remaining well despite the miserable situation between her parents.

Family 15. Edward Brown

History

Edward, aged 24, was born in the UK and is of African–Caribbean ethnicity. He lives with his mother and brother George, who is aged 18.

The parents separated when Edward was aged 10 and he then lived with his father and grandmother. He passed 5 GCSEs but failed 2 A levels. He was then accepted for a course of study at a higher education college in Trinidad. He attended there for 1 year while living with an aunt.

He returned to the UK to start a course in economics at university and moved in with mother. Both his father and mother are local council employees. During the 2 years he spent at university he became increasingly isolated.

He was first admitted to a psychiatric unit at age 21 complaining of abdominal pains, low mood and little energy. No physical cause was found for his pain and a diagnosis of depression was made. He was discharged home after 3 weeks.

He was readmitted a year later after behaving strangely in a shop. He again complained of abdominal pains. His mother discharged him after a few hours, but he was readmitted some months later with the same symptoms. This time he remained in hospital for 8 months and a referral was made for family therapy. The family missed many sessions and were discharged from the clinic after several months.

Recently Edward has been prescribed a novel antipsychotic, but his adherence has been irregular and his attendance at the clinic erratic. He has joined a number of adult education classes and is keen to return to university. He is able to process information well, but is physically slow and is still complaining of abdominal pains. He has difficulty getting up in the morning.

Recently he has been assigned a council flat but has not moved in yet. He has difficulty travelling by public transport but can drive a car. He used to enjoy playing football but no longer does so.

Presenting problems

Mother put a lot of pressure on a college to accept him for a degree course and he has been offered a place to study politics and economics. However, he complains that the area in which the college is located is very racist.

The therapist saw mother together with Edward for the first time. She noted that Edward becomes very passive in mother's presence and echoes her statements. Should he return to higher education or is this unrealistic? How can Edward be helped to move into his own flat?

Formulation

Following his parents' separation, Edward lived with his father for several years but after his return from Trinidad he moved in with his mother. It is not clear whether these changes of residence were his choice or were dictated by his parents. Either way he must have developed divided loyalties. His father's emotional attitude to him is as yet unknown and he needs to be brought into the picture. His mother is evidently overinvolved with him, since he becomes very passive in her presence and allows her to dominate him although he is 24 years old. Her behaviour in discharging him prematurely from the psychiatric ward is further evidence of overinvolvement.

Another unknown factor is how far Edward's desire to return to university is driven by his mother's ambition for him, given that she pressurised the college to accept him. His objection that the college is in a very racist area does not ring true and indicates ambivalence at the least.

Edward's failure to move into his flat suggests that he has difficulty leaving his mother and is quite dependent on her. Both his dependence and her overinvolvement will need to be the focus of family work. His younger brother George should be recruited to help with this endeavour, since he may be able to voice an objective view of the relationship between Edward and mother.

Supervisor's suggestions

1. Organise a joint meeting with mother, Edward and George.
2. At a later stage try to see father together with Edward.

Follow-up

12 months

Edward started at college and did well in the first year, passing seven of eight subjects. However, he relapsed shortly after the end of year exam, showing what a strain studying is for him. He had several changes of medication during the academic year and had been hearing voices. The last change of medication was just before the exams, in retrospect an unwise time to prescribe a drug he had never received before. He has also gained weight.

He has been irregular in attending the clinic and in taking his medication. Mother phones and complains about the service.

Edward returned to college for the next academic year starting in October. One month later his grandmother died. She had helped to look after him when his parents separated. He stopped attending college then and said he had been low since she died.

During this period George left school at age 18 and he has been doing vocational training.

Edward cooks for himself. He is mostly monosyllabic and socialises mainly with older family members. Mother attends Edward's clinic appointments irregularly but accompanied him at his last visit. She was more subdued than before and said Edward should take more responsibility for himself. She was offered a session with the therapist on her own and she welcomed it.

Edward has had three sessions of cognitive therapy. He did not like the experience and his therapist thinks it brings out his psychopathology.

He has contacted the disability officer on his own initiative.

Supervisor's suggestions

1. Mother's critical attitude to the services is typical of overinvolved relatives, who are often rivalrous with professional carers. However, she was eager to see the therapist on her own. This provides an opportunity to congratulate her on her care of Edward and to reinforce her desire to see him become more independent.

2. Try to discover more from mother about the circumstances of the separation and why the boys stayed with father. Also determine the extent of father's involvement with Edward.

3. Although Edward can cope with the demands of a university course intellectually, the emotional strain puts him at risk for another relapse. Prepare him for possible academic failure and encourage him to consider an alternative career. He will need to be helped with grief work over the loss of his academic aspirations.

14 months

Edward is still hearing voices but cannot make out the words. They only trouble him a bit. He was invited to attend a clinic for cognitive therapy from a psychologist.

Mother has become more engaged with staff: she was seen at home by the therapist. Father had custody of the boys when they separated, as she was in a refuge. This suggests that her husband physically abused her. Father wanted to be seen as a professional carer and was embarrassed at being offered help. She reported that father denied her access to Edward from age 10 to 14 and asserted that father rejected Edward when George was born. However, Edward goes to football matches with father at weekends. Father is a referee and Edward acts as a linesman.

Mother was not keen to see the therapist together with Edward. At their last meeting George was hovering as if he wanted to be asked in.

Supervisor's suggestions

1. Mother's account of the separation is puzzling. If she was in a refuge because of father's violence, there was no justification for

him to have legal custody of the boys. Furthermore, if there was a legal separation, mother would have been granted access to her sons. It might clarify matters to hear father's side of the story.
2. Invite George personally to come to a meeting with mother or else with Edward.

16 months

Mother is still very critical of services: shouting and screaming about them. Edward has just finished a year at university and is more psychotic than ever. He has been offered clozapine but refuses blood tests. He has been sent an appointment for further cognitive therapy and is agreeable.

Father is unpredictable: he asks Edward to be a linesman at a match at half an hour's notice. He has given Edward a book on schizophrenia.

It is difficult to talk to Edward about emotional issues because he is not forthcoming. However, he has revealed that he feels that George is disrespectful to him.

Supervisor's suggestion
Try to meet with George and Edward together without mother. Raise the issue of the boys' separation from mother for 4 years while they lived with father.

18 months

Edward has been working full-time at a newsagent but has now stopped. He is still muttering to himself. He has been referred to a drop-in centre which offers advice and counselling.

The therapist met with George for the first time a few weeks ago.

Supervisor's suggestion
Try to arrange a meeting with father.

21 months

Mother now says she does not want Edward living with her any more. She wants him to move to his own flat. She is aware of him being understimulated.

Supervisor's suggestion
He might benefit from attending a hearing voices group.

Commentary

In Family 14 the parents shared a home but nothing else. In this family the parents lived apart and did not communicate, but father still had contact with his sons and exerted a strong influence. The story of the separation from mother's point of view contained inconsistencies and it

75

did not prove possible to meet with father to hear his version. It is likely that the sons were as confused about the real events as was the therapist. Despite efforts to meet with more than one member of this family at a time, the therapist never managed to achieve this. Their resistance to joint meetings suggests that the members have difficulty in feeling like a family and communicating with each other. Father's action in giving Edward a book on schizophrenia instead of talking to him about his illness is an illustration of this.

Despite these difficulties and mother's extremely critical attitude to the services offered, the therapist was able to form a working relationship with her. Through this, mother's overinvolvement diminished to the point where she was keen for Edward to move into his own flat. He was able to cook for himself, but would probably need help with other aspects of independent living to manage the flat on his own. If he did live by himself there is a danger of his becoming very isolated. Members of his extended family and his brother George would need to be encouraged to provide a supportive network for him.

Edward struggled to continue with his studies despite persistent positive and negative symptoms of schizophrenia that were not fully controlled by medication. Although he was able cope with the demands of the course intellectually, he relapsed shortly after he completed the exams. It is advisable for people with this degree of vulnerability to postpone the completion of their studies for a few years until their illness has stabilised. This entails the mourning of their lost expectations, which Edward did not manage to do with the therapist. Nevertheless he did take on an undemanding full-time job for a while, indicating an awareness of the need to scale down his aspirations.

CHAPTER 6

Dysfunctional families

Dysfunctional family is a term used by family therapists to indicate severe disruption of family roles and relationships. The appearance of a psychotic illness in a family member can stress relationships and alter roles but rarely produces the severity of disturbance seen in dysfunctional families. Thus many of the problems evident to the therapists who are seeing a patient living in a dysfunctional family pre-date the onset of the psychosis. It is important for the therapists to make a clear distinction between the problems stemming from the patient's illness and those inherent in the family, even though the latter will inevitably affect the patient. In these families it is common to find violations of inter-generational boundaries, sometimes even inappropriate sexual relation-ships. The therapists may find it essential to address some of the family's dysfunctional problems in order to enable the patient to progress.

Family 16. Ann Harcourt

History

Ann is aged 22 and lives with her parents and a sister, Frances, who is aged 19. Father is a travelling salesman who is home every evening and at weekends. Mother is a doctor's receptionist. Frances has just finished high school.

At age 16 Ann was referred to a psychologist by her school. Her parents were not informed. She continued seeing the psychologist as an out-patient until the age of 18 when he arranged her admission to an adolescent unit. The parents were still kept in ignorance but Frances was told by Ann and sworn to secrecy. Ann stayed in this unit for 1 year, was diagnosed as suffering from paranoid schizophrenia and was treated with clozapine. She was then discharged to a sheltered home for adolescents. In the home she talked to her case manager about sexual abuse from her parents, her sister and other adults. The case manager was alarmed and sent a letter to a social worker reporting the allegations. The social worker contacted the family and showed them the letter. They were very shocked by Ann's accusations and by learning that she had been in psychiatric care for 6 years without them knowing. The social worker interviewed the parents and sister and decided that the accusations were delusional.

The family was in crisis and contacted a community psychiatric nurse. This therapist saw only the parents. Father was very angry with Ann about her accusation against him. The parents attended six sessions of psychoeducation in a relatives' group. They accepted that Ann was ill but thought it was because of contact with other disturbed young people. Mother felt intensely guilty about not having helped her daughter.

Presenting problems

How can the parents be reconciled with Ann after she has deceived them for so many years? How can they be helped to accept the nature of her illness?

Formulation

This family lives in a country where the rights of a person over the age of 16 override the obligation to inform the parents about any medical treatment given. Nevertheless, it is necessary to question why Ann felt it necessary to conceal her psychiatric problems from her parents, although revealing them to her sister. This suggests either that mental illness is heavily stigmatised in this family or that there are many taboo subjects which cannot be talked about. Sexuality may be one of these and could explain the content of Ann's delusion of being sexually abused by family members. Meetings with the family should focus on what is safe to talk about and what is unsafe.

The parents' belief that Ann's illness is due to contact with disturbed young people is quite common in the initial stages of coming to terms with the diagnosis of schizophrenia. The first response is usually shock, followed by disbelief and a search for alternative explanations, including street drugs and mixing with a 'bad crowd'. The therapist needs to be patient and sensitive to the parents' inability to take in the official diagnosis. It can take many months before they are able to accept that the illness is schizophrenia, and some parents never reach this stage.

Supervisor's suggestion

At this early stage in the education of the family about schizophrenia, it is inadvisable to challenge the parents' view of the causation of Ann's illness. The therapist can repeat the message about the biological basis of schizophrenia without negating the family's belief. Instead, the emphasis should be on the family doing their best to support their daughter. Hold a meeting with the whole family to explore how they can help Ann to recover.

Follow-up

1 month

One session was held by two therapists in the family home, attended by the parents and Frances. Mother and father did not want Ann to be there. Frances told them she knew about Ann's contact with the psychologist. Mother cried and Frances was angry with mother but was not asked the reason for this.

Supervisor's suggestions

The parents are obviously very upset and angry about Ann's failure to confide in them and her accusations of sexual abuse by them and by Frances. Their response is to exclude her from the sessions. This may be to protect her from their anger or themselves from further damaging accusations in the presence of the therapists. However, it is noteworthy that the therapists did not explore the cause of Frances' expression of anger in the session. They are being affected by this family's prohibition of the discussion of emotional issues, which is likely to be the main reason they do not want Ann to join them. The therapists need to gently probe the individual members' emotional responses to Ann's revelations and to help them feel safe to express them.

3 months

The therapists have been meeting with the three family members every 2 weeks. In the sessions mother and father always agree about everything: there is never any open disagreement. Frances is more outspoken and, although hurt and puzzled by her sister's accusation, is prepared to accept that it stemmed from her psychiatric illness and to forgive her. Eventually the family agreed that Ann should join the sessions. This was not to tackle the emotional disturbances she is the centre of, but ostensibly because Ann wanted to go on holiday together with her family and they needed to come to a decision.

Supervisor's suggestions

1. The unnaturally perfect agreement between the parents on every issue appears to be 'pseudo-mutuality' (Wynne *et al*, 1958), a situation in which any disagreement cannot be tolerated and is therefore concealed by a tacit convention to present a united front. This is probably the source of Ann's secrecy about her teenage emotional disturbance that eventually developed into schizophrenia. The therapists have no brief to address the parents' intolerance of

dissent and anyway they face such a strong coalition that any intervention would be likely to fail. Instead the therapists should focus on strengthening the alliance between Ann and Frances.

2. A holiday together offers the chance of a reconciliation and should be encouraged. It will require some negotiation between the family members on how long it should be and the allocation of bedrooms. Preferably Ann should have a bedroom of her own to which she can retire when she finds social interaction stressful. The most stressful vacation for a person with schizophrenia is a caravan holiday with the family, which allows no means of escape.

4 months

The first full family session occurred. Ann sat at the end of the table and father sat as far away from her as possible. He appeared to be very angry but was not expressing it. Frances sat next to Ann and was supportive of her. Mother was often on the verge of tears. It was agreed that they would spend 1 week on holiday by the sea and that Ann and Frances would each have a bedroom.

6 months

The family went on holiday together with Ann. They managed to control any conflict by avoiding leaving father and Ann alone together. Now father is a bit less angry but mother is still feeling guilty.

Supervisor's suggestions

1. Mother appears to be more open in expressing her feelings than father. Attempt to meet with mother on her own to allow her to express her guilt and to reassure her that she could not have caused Ann's illness. It could help reduce her sense of guilt to attend an ongoing carers' group with or without her husband.

2. Arrange to meet with the two sisters to emphasise the inter-generational boundary and to explore the possibility of Frances taking Ann to age-appropriate events.

Commentary

The silence in this family over any disturbing matters led to Ann's secrecy about her need for psychological help. The therapists also felt constrained by the fact that emotional issues were taboo, which impaired their ability to work effectively at first. One therapist felt they should have opened up the area of unexpressed emotions but the other thought it was too risky. A useful strategy for dealing with this dilemma is for the therapists to have a discussion in front of the family about their own disagreement over this issue. This would not only open up the issue of concealment, but also demonstrate to the family that two people in a partnership can disagree openly without drastic consequences. The therapeutic team sometimes mirrors the family's emotional conflicts unconsciously and needs to become aware of this process in order to tackle the problem at source (Berkowitz & Leff, 1984).

The content of Ann's delusions indicates that she is in conflict over her sexuality and needs to discuss the issues with her therapist. The family's silence about emotional issues presumably also extended to sexual feelings and interests in the daughters. Ann probably had to deal with her emerging sexuality on her own until she was referred to a psychologist. Her emotional disturbance was a direct threat to the parental defence of mutual agreement not to allow any conflicts to surface. Consequently she concealed it until they were forced to confront it by her delusional accusations. They then dealt with it by banning her from family sessions at first and then keeping her as far away from father as possible. This family apparently believes that if Ann and her father are allowed to get too close something unspeakable will happen. Is it violence or sex they fear?

Ann's best option is probably to keep in touch with her parents through her sister. She has already shown trust in Frances by confiding in her earlier in the illness. Frances seems to be robust enough to act as liaison between Ann and their parents. Ann is already in a supportive environment in the sheltered home and this is probably her best route to independent living.

Family 17. Paul Goodwin

History

Paul is aged 26 and lives with his father Howard, who is a documentary film maker, his mother Caroline, who works in a boutique, and his sister Roberta, aged 20. The parents were hippies and disregarded Paul's disturbed behaviour as a youth. He performed poorly at school, and in his teens decided to live as a squatter and adopted an alternative lifestyle.

At age 21 Paul made his first contact with psychiatric services when he attended an emergency clinic with a panic attack. One year later he developed disorganised thinking and delusions that he could change the world. He was admitted to a psychiatric hospital and given a diagnosis of schizophrenia. He continued on antipsychotic medication for 1 year and attended a day hospital intermittently. He had continuous delusions of catastrophe and experienced auditory hallucinations. His affect was blunted. He locked himself in his room all day, but his parents were ambivalent about recognising that he was ill.

Another crisis occurred 6 months later and he was admitted for 4 months. He was tried on various medications with little improvement.

Every time he went home for the weekend he returned to hospital in a worse state.

On his discharge to the day hospital family work was started. Father was hopeless and critical of Paul, complaining that he did not have his feet on the ground. Paul had begun painting rapidly and frequently. His parents do not recognise the value of his art and are critical of his painting. They are always entering Paul's room asking 'Are you allright? Is there anything I can do for you?'

The family never eat together. Roberta sometimes eats with Paul but he eats very fast and 'like an animal', which makes her nervous. In the session the parents did not interact and there was no eye contact between them.

Paul admires father's knowledge of music and musicians. He is also fond of Roberta and he enjoys cooking.

Presenting problems

In an attempt to strengthen Paul's relationships with the family members, the two therapists suggested that Paul shares music with father, shares cooking with mother and shares the computer with Roberta. Father and Paul went out to buy CDs together early on a Saturday morning. However, mother was not able to let Paul share cooking because 'he makes too much disorder'.

How can his parents be helped to accept the nature of his illness? Can Paul be integrated into his family? Can they be encouraged to appreciate his creativity?

Formulation

The Goodwin family presents a variety of different problems. The parents have not abandoned the hippy culture they embraced in their youth, and view Paul's disturbed behaviour as the manifestation of a free spirit. In contradiction to this stance, they dismiss his paintings, which probably belong to the genre of 'Outsider Art', a growing field increasingly recognised and valued by art critics.

The family is also fragmented: they do not share meals, the parents did not interact when seen together and Paul is isolated from the individual members, except possibly his sister. Father is openly critical of his son and both parents are overinvolved, as shown by their constant intrusions into his room with expressions of concern. The observation by the staff of the day hospital that Paul's mental state was always worse when he returned from a stay with the family is indicative of high expressed emotion in the home environment.

The therapists' attempt to strengthen Paul's relationships with his relatives seemed to bear fruit with father, but mother was intolerant of his disorganised behaviour. The parents' lack of reciprocity and the weak alliance between them provide the therapists with little to build on. When parents are incapable of cooperating, they are inevitably poor at tackling the problems posed by the care of a relative with schizophrenia.

It will be important to modify father's critical attitude and to attempt to reduce both parents' overinvolvement in order to protect Paul from the emotional stress to which he is exposed at home. Educational sessions should be held to try to modify the parents' attitude to Paul's disturbed behaviour. An acceptance of his psychiatric illness is likely to ameliorate father's criticism of his son. It is also important to give the parents hope of an improvement in Paul's condition. The therapists should stress that his creativity is a strength on which his recovery can be based. Furthermore, it would help to boost Paul's self-esteem if his parents could be induced to value his artwork. As with Family 16, the approach most likely to succeed is to build on Paul's relationship with his sister. She is the only family member who tries to eat with him.

Supervisor's suggestions

1. Hold educational sessions with the family, including Paul.
2. Find a catalogue of Outsider Art and show it to the family.
3. See Paul and Roberta together and explore their mutual interests.

Follow-up

1 month

Paul had an exhibition of his paintings in a bar and sold three of them for a considerable sum. At the time he was improving mentally and attending the day hospital regularly. No family member came to the exhibition. Following this he became worse again, stopped attending the day hospital and gave up painting.

3 months

The therapists held a number of educational sessions with the whole family. Father became less critical and less despondent about Paul's future. Paul wanted to stop the sessions and complained that the therapists were trying to normalise the family. He said he preferred them to exist separately: father with his music, mother in the kitchen and Roberta on her own. His choice is to be isolated. He stood up when stating this opinion and was emphatic, which made the therapists anxious.

Supervisor's suggestion

Paul communicated to the therapists his anxiety about the family coming together as a unit. His delusions of catastrophe indicate that he fears his own destructiveness and is trying to protect his family by keeping them separate. On the other hand he is capable of directing his fierce energy into the creative act of painting. There is a resemblance to van Gogh, most of whose paintings were produced in the space of a few years and who ended up mutilating and then destroying himself. Paul's intense anxiety has to be respected. Continue to hold sessions with the parents and Roberta, without Paul, but give him the option of returning to the sessions when he feels able to.

4 months

During the next few sessions it became apparent that the parents were approaching each other, doing things together and sharing interests.

5 months

Paul rejoined the sessions after a few weeks but did not participate. His self-care had deteriorated and he was not attending the day hospital, but he had resumed painting.

6 months

After two more sessions the parents said they did not want any more meetings. Since then, mother phones every month, and has asked for more therapy.

Commentary

Initially it did not seem likely that the therapists could improve the relationship between the parents, but they succeeded in bringing them closer together and helping them to enjoy each other's company. Furthermore, they enabled father to moderate his anger towards his son. Although we would judge these changes in the family environment to be beneficial, Paul was disturbed by them and pleaded for a return to the previous situation of fragmentation.

Paul has intense anxiety about his destructiveness, as expressed through his delusions about creating chaos in the whole world. He is fearful of destroying his family if they get too close and believes he has to keep them apart. His feared destructiveness is compensated for by his creativity, which has received recognition from the public, if not his parents. He has also started making pottery at the day hospital, although there is no tutor there for this medium.

The parents eventually asked for the meetings to cease, although the therapists wished to continue. The parents' reason for withdrawing from the therapy was quite different from Paul's. Quite often when a family becomes aware that they are changing, they become alarmed at the process and where it will lead. They may respond by dismissing the therapists. However, once change has begun it develops its own momentum. Mother's regular phone calls to the therapists after their dismissal and her request for more therapy is an illustration of this.

For the future it will be important for the therapists to make a clear distinction between the problematic aspects of the parents' relationship and Paul's problems stemming from his illness. They will need to clarify whether the parents want couple therapy. Paul's creativity should be nurtured through his painting and pottery. He would benefit from an individual teacher, who might be able to help him use his art as a way of communicating his anxieties.

CHAPTER 7

Unresolved past trauma

Sexual abuse in childhood and other traumas, which lead to a sense of shame or intense anxiety if dwelt upon, are often concealed from the person's partner. If the individual develops a psychotic illness later in life, the earlier trauma can be reactivated and may reappear in the form of psychotic experiences or apparently baseless guilt and self-reproach. The way the individual copes with traumatic events influences the later emergence of psychotic disturbances. An internet survey of 1202 people found paranoid thoughts to occur regularly in one-third of the sample (Freeman *et al*, 2005). More intense paranoid ideation was associated with negative attitudes to the expression of emotion, feeling inferior to others and not accepted by them, and behaving submissively. Therapeutic interventions that are likely to help include encouragement to talk about the paranoia, increasing the person's self-esteem, help in negotiating relationships with others, and developing feelings of control over the situation (Chadwick *et al*, 1996). The patient is also likely to need additional personal therapy to help deal with the past trauma and to facilitate disclosure to the partner.

Family 18. Albertina Kidd

History

Albertina is aged 58 and suffers from a recurrent depressive psychosis. In the past 6 years she has taken five overdoses, each of which necessitated an admission. When depressed she believes people are watching her and bugging her phone. She was born in Jamaica and came to the UK at age 22. She was trained in nursing and worked as a night sister for 20 years. As a result of her depressive episodes she was retired on the grounds of ill health. She suffers from non-insulin-dependent diabetes, pulmonary embolism and osteoarthritis, and has been fitted with a pacemaker. Her depressive episodes started with worry about her physical health, financial worries and a sense of guilt. Her guilt is centred around the feeling that she should be working. She believes she is being followed by members of the Department of Social Security. She has been attending a psychologist for cognitive therapy, which is helping.

Her husband Henri is aged 60 and came to the UK from Martinique. He has a degree in chemistry and was studying up to 3 years ago. He used to lecture but no longer works. They have two sons, who are quite supportive. One has moved away, the other has a girlfriend and lives at home.

When Albertina becomes ill, Henri thinks she should pull herself together. He is a rigid man who is overpowering and takes over meetings. He uses pseudo-psychological terms. His mother told him she hated him and wished he had never been born. Albertina reports that 'He picks at things to put her down'. He sees the female therapist as forming a relationship with his wife from which he is excluded. They live off her nursing pension and she does all the housework.

Presenting problems

How can Henri be persuaded to become more understanding of and supportive to his wife? How can Albertina's guilt about not working be dealt with?

Formulation

Albertina has a serious psychiatric illness and a complex of physical illnesses. These are more than sufficient reason for her to be unable to work. Her guilt therefore has no rational basis and must stem from other causes. This needs to be explored with her in individual sessions.

Henri contributes nothing to the family economy, neither income nor housework, and this should be tackled. However, his rigidity may impede efforts to change his lifestyle. The roles for men and women in the Caribbean tend to be more clearly demarcated than in the UK and this will compound the difficulty of achieving change.

Henri is critical of Albertina when she is depressed and this has been shown to predict relapses (Miklowitz *et al*, 1988). Their problematic relationship needs to be addressed in sessions with the couple, focusing on how Henri reacts to her depression and how Albertina responds to his criticism (Jones & Asen, 2000). The two sons could prove useful allies in commenting on their parents' relationship and in providing their mother with additional emotional and practical support.

Supervisor's suggestions

1. Encourage husband and wife to go out together to enjoy themselves. The couple should be encouraged to think back to when they were first married and to choose an outing that gave them pleasure then.

2. Ask Henri to think of something he could do in the house to help his wife.

3. Reframe his criticism in terms of caring and ask the couple to say one thing they like about one another.

4. Invite the sons to a joint family meeting.

5. Ensure that one of the two therapists is a man to facilitate forming an alliance with Henri, who feels shut out of the relationship between his wife and the female therapist.

Follow-up

2 months

A meeting was held with Albertina and Henri and a male and female therapist. Before the meeting Albertina asked Henri to help her tidy up and he became so angry that he frightened her. His general practitioner has prescribed antidepressants for him in the past. He used to confide in the general practitioner but he died recently.

Albertina's family blame Henri for his treatment of her. Henri says she is now better and more assertive and he feels he has no more reason to stay with her.

Supervisor's suggestion

It is not clear how serious Henri is about leaving Albertina. In order to explore this the therapists should ask the couple to discuss what they need from each other and how each can satisfy the other's needs.

4 months

Henri went to Martinique for a visit and Albertina became very depressed a few days later and took an overdose. She was admitted on Christmas Eve. It emerged for the first time that Albertina was raped at age 19 at Christmas time. The therapists intended to explore it with her, but the discussion had to be postponed because of the dominance of her current psychiatric symptoms. Albertina had voiced her concerns about the rape to her primary nurse on the ward.

A meeting was arranged by the therapists with the two sons. Their parents had protected them from knowledge of Albertina's psychiatric illness and they were quite shocked. They felt they had not done enough to help.

Supervisor's suggestions

1. Albertina's revelation of the rape, which she had kept secret for 40 years, explains her abiding sense of guilt, which previously appeared irrational. She needs individual sessions with the female therapist to allow her to express her feelings about it.

2. The sons are very willing to help their mother and should be recruited to give support.

10 months

The sons coped during her admission and took a leading role in Henri's absence. She was discharged after 2 months, but became depressed again a few weeks later and took another overdose. It took a month of daily visits to re-establish her on her medication regime. The female therapist tried to convene regular meetings between the couple, herself and the male therapist, but after two sessions Henri phoned her to complain that he felt very criticised and refused to attend again.

Supervisor's suggestions
1. Henri is obviously very sensitive and interprets requests to change as criticism. His response is a confirmation of his rigidity and indicates that there is no point in trying to continue with joint meetings. He could benefit from having individual sessions with his own therapist.
2. Suggest to Albertina that she considers taking on voluntary work as a way of repaying her financial benefits from the state.

12 months

Albertina was fine until a few days ago, when Henri told a friend about her suicide attempt and elaborated it incorrectly. The friend told Albertina and now Henri won't let the friend in the house any more. Albertina now says she wants to leave him but cannot afford to move out.

Their son who lives with them helps with the situation at home. He provides her with company. Henri does not speak to her for weeks at a time. Albertina has started attending a sewing group run by her therapist.

14 months

Albertina was admitted 2 weeks ago for serious suicidal thoughts. She had stopped eating. She is still paranoid about people in the street saying she is a burden on the state. She has started to do voluntary work at a day centre.

Henri has started meeting with a male psychologist.

18 months

Albertina is doing well at the sewing group, making her own clothes.

22 months

Albertina is quite well. Henri is well engaged with the psychologist and asked him to tell them how to manage Albertina.

24 months

Albertina deteriorated 2 months ago. She is now improving and avoided admission.

Commentary

The Kidd family exhibit a number of the problems discussed above. Albertina has significant physical illnesses in addition to her psychiatric condition; she and Henri come from different cultures, hers anglophone, his francophone; they have a disturbed relationship and each has threatened to leave the other at some time; and important events have been concealed from some family members: her rape from Henri and her mental illness from their sons. The concealment was prompted by shame and embarrassment and led to adverse consequences. Albertina was left with a feeling of guilt, which was transmuted into a delusion, and she was denied the support of her sons, which they would have given willingly.

The meetings between the two therapists and the couple were not sustainable because of Henri's sensitivity, but he was able to engage with a male psychologist in individual sessions, which he began to make use of. It is not clear whether Albertina was able to work through her feelings about the rape with her therapist, but her paranoid delusion did not disappear. An alternative strategy was tried of encouraging her to undertake voluntary work, and she engaged well with this, in addition to joining a sewing group. She also received more support from the son who lives at home. These changes had the effect of enlarging her support network and giving her the feeling of contributing to other people's well-being, which she must have had during her career as a nurse.

Although the changes in her social environment and personal satisfaction did not prevent her from having a further episode of depression, for the first time in 8 years she was able to manage without being admitted to hospital. For the future it is important for the psychologist to continue working with Henri on coping strategies he could use when Albertina begins to show signs of depression.

CHAPTER 8

Exploitative carer

Although the vast majority of carers have the best of intentions towards the patient, exceptionally a carer may take advantage of the patient's vulnerability for their own benefit. The unscrupulous carer will then see the professionals as trying to displace them from their role. Therapists need to exercise great care in working with the patient to decrease their vulnerability without alienating them.

Family 19. Adele Ojede

History

Adele is aged 30 and was born in Nigeria. She suffers from paranoid delusions about being mistaken for another woman who is mentally ill, while she herself is sane. Her mother left her father with eight children when Adele was aged 9. The children were fostered and Adele has a long history of being in care as a child. Some of her siblings now live locally. Her father now suffers from dementia and is cared for in a nursing home.

Her mother called in Adele's brother Lester because she visited Adele's flat and found it in a mess. Lester found the flat in a shambles and contacted the social worker with the complaint that his sister had been neglected by the services. He moved into her flat and asserted that he was her full-time carer. He claims to be a criminologist. Adele says he does not stay overnight as he has a pregnant girlfriend. A community psychiatric nurse went to visit her flat. Adele would not see her and refused contact with the services. She was then admitted involuntarily.

After Adele's discharge a continual series of complaints about the community psychiatric nurse was received from Lester. A meeting with Adele and Lester was arranged. It became very confrontational: Adele did not want to engage with the services and left the meeting. Lester eventually apologised. He has joined the local carers' organisation. He continued to call three times a day and said he was sacking the community psychiatric nurse.

Presenting problems

Lester has split up with his partner, who is the tenant of the flat they were sharing, and he has moved in with Adele. He is now pressing for her to be allocated a two-bedroom flat on the grounds that he is her carer. It appears that Lester is acting more out of self-interest than from a genuine feeling of concern for his sister. How can he be disengaged from Adele? How can she be persuaded to adhere to her medication and follow-up visits?

Formulation

Adele comes from a large sibship of eight, suggesting that this is a traditional family. However, the fact that mother separated from her husband and left all the children with him is far from traditional and led to Adele spending years in care. A history of years of separation from parents during childhood has been identified as a risk factor for schizophrenia in minority ethnic groups in the UK (Mallett *et al*, 2002).

The siblings in a traditional family are expected to care for an ill relative, and Lester's behaviour can be seen as appropriate in this context. His constant criticism of the services is typical of an over-involved relative who fears being displaced from their role by the professional carers. On the other hand, there is a definite advantage for him to stay in Adele's flat now he has separated from his partner, and there may be an exploitative element in his behaviour.

Supervisor's suggestion

If concern for his sister is his overriding motivation, he will cooperate with the services to ensure that she gets the treatment she needs. Use this as a test of his intentions.

Follow-up

2 months

Adele has been admitted to hospital again. She says she does not want Lester to be her carer or come to her flat. Lester has now gone back to his girlfriend, who has just had her baby.

3 months

Lester came to the ward and took Adele home for overnight leave but failed to bring her back. She is now back on the ward. Lester kept complaining about the therapist. She brought in another colleague but Lester would not let her into the flat either. Adele is not in agreement with Lester's accusations against her therapist and has dismissed him as her carer. The therapist tried to contact Adele's mother and sisters but Lester blocked her.

6 months

Lester disappeared for a while, probably having his time taken up with the new baby. He was seen by the social worker the previous week and said that he wants to be Adele's carer again.

Commentary

As events unfolded it became clear that Lester was not acting in his sister's best interests. She herself made it clear that she did not welcome his activities on her behalf. Her interests need to be protected by the services and this is best done by her therapist forming an alliance with her. However, the fact that she had to be admitted involuntarily is an impediment to the development of a trusting relationship. It seems sensible for the therapist to obtain Adele's permission to contact her mother in order to explain the situation to her, given that the mother called in Lester in the first place. He may feel he has his mother's authority to override Adele's wishes. Mother would need to be educated about Adele's illness to gain her cooperation in telling her son to keep his distance.

CHAPTER 9

Postscript

The reader will have noticed that some of my suggested interventions were taken up by the therapists and produced the intended changes. Others were implemented but had no obvious effect, and some were not utilised at all. At no time did I insist that the therapists carry out the interventions I felt to be appropriate. I did not meet with any of these families, so that the therapists were in a better position than I was to judge what was likely to be acceptable to their clients. Sometimes therapists feel inhibited about trying a specific intervention with a particular family, and this may reveal an emotional effect the family is having on them. I was always alert to this possibility and would bring it to the therapists' attention if I thought it was operating. It should not be viewed negatively as an impediment to progress, but as a valuable source of information about the emotional problems of the family. At other times the therapists had no opportunity to introduce an intervention, either because the family members concerned did not attend the sessions, or because the family's circumstances had changed.

Supervision of family work is essential, either from an experienced therapist or from one's peer group, because the work is emotionally taxing and sometimes faces the therapists with extremely difficult problems, as illustrated by the families presented here. The more minds that are brought to bear on a problem, the more likely it is that a creative solution will emerge. No supervisor is omniscient or infallible, and suggested interventions should be viewed as experiments that might or might not succeed. There is no crucial moment in work with families caring for a person with a psychotic illness. What fails at one point in time can succeed later. With long-standing illnesses there is no such thing as a missed opportunity to intervene. There will always be another chance to try out an intervention at a later date. It is important to be flexible and not to be disappointed when an intervention has no apparent effect.

Sometimes therapists feel like giving up when faced by a difficult family that seems to be stuck. This is another reason why a support group for therapists engaged in this work is essential. Members of a group can point out that the family's hopelessness can readily affect the therapist, but that the origin of the lack of hope lies in the family and not in the therapist. They can support the therapist by brainstorming on ways to help the family out of their rut. This should encourage the therapist to think constructively about the family and to tackle their pessimism. In this work the most valuable contribution a therapist can make is to give the families and the patients hope. If you do nothing else, your efforts will have been worthwhile.

References

Ball, R. A., Moore, E. & Kuipers, E. (1992) Expressed emotion in community care staff: a comparison of patient outcome in a nine month follow-up of two hostels. *Social Psychiatry and Psychiatric Epidemiology*, **27**, 35–39.

Bateson, G., Jackson, D. D., Haley, J., *et al* (1956) Towards a theory of schizophrenia. *Behavioral Science*, **1**, 251–264.

Berkowitz, R. & Leff, J. (1984) Clinical teams reflect family dysfunction. *Journal of Family Therapy*, **6**, 78–89.

Chadwick, P. (1995) *Understanding Paranoia*. London: Thorsons.

Chadwick, P. D. J., Birchwood, M. J. & Trower, P. (1996) *Cognitive Therapy for Delusions, Voices and Paranoia*. Chichester: Wiley.

Cooklin, A. (2004) Talking with children and their understanding of mental illness. In *Parental Psychiatric Disorder: Distressed Parents and their Families* (2nd edn) (eds M. Göpfert, J. Webster & M. V. Seeman), pp. 292–305. Cambridge: Cambridge University Press.

Department of Health (2002) *Mental Health Policy Implementation Guide: Dual Diagnosis Good Practice Guide*. London: Department of Health.

Fearon, P., Jones, P. B., Kennedy, N., *et al* (2004) Raised incidence of psychosis in all migrant groups in South London, Nottingham and Bristol: the AESOP Study. *Schizophrenia Research*, **67**, (suppl. 1), 15.

Freeman, D., Garety, P. A., Bebbington, P. E., *et al* (2005) Psychological investigation of the structure of paranoia in a non-clinical population. *British Journal of Psychiatry*, **186**, 427–435.

Hammersley, P., Dias, A., Todd, D., *et al* (2003) Childhood trauma and hallucinations in bipolar affective disorder: preliminary investigation. *British Journal of Psychiatry*, **182**, 543–547.

Jablensky, A., Sartorius, N., Ernberg, G., *et al* (1992) Schizophrenia manifestations, incidence and course in different cultures. A World Health Organization ten-country study. *Psychological Medicine Monograph Supplement*, **20**. Cambridge: Cambridge University Press.

Janssen, I., Krabbendam, L., Bak, M., *et al* (2004) Childhood abuse as a risk factor for psychotic experiences. *Acta Psychiatrica Scandinavica*, **109**, 38–45.

Jones, E. & Asen, E. (2000) *Systemic Couple Therapy and Depression*. London: Karnac.

Koenigsberg, H., Klausner, E. Pelicano, D., *et al* (1993) Expressed emotion and glucose control in insulin-dependent diabetes mellitus. *American Journal of Psychiatry*, **150**, 1114–1115.

Kuipers, E., Leff, J. & Lam, D. (2002) *Family Work for Schizophrenia: A Practical Guide* (2nd edn). London: Gaskell.

Lappin, J. M., Dazzan, P., Morgan, K., *et al* (2003) Length of untreated psychotic symptoms and effects on brain structure in the AESOP first-onset psychosis study (abstract). XII Biennial Winter Workshop on Schizophrenia, Davos. *Schizophrenia Research*, **67** (suppl. 1), 97.

Larsen, T. K., McGlashan, T. H., Johannessen, J. O., *et al* (2001) Shortened duration of untreated first episode of psychosis: changes in patient characteristics at treatment. *American Journal of Psychiatry*, **158**, 1917–1919.

Leff, J. P. (1968) Perceptual phenomena and personality in sensory deprivation. *British Journal of Psychiatry*, **114**, 1499–1508.

Leff, J. & Vaughn, C. (1985) *Expressed Emotion in Families: Its Significance for Mental Illness*. New York: Guilford.

Leff, J., Kuipers, L., Berkowitz, R., *et al* (1982) A controlled trial of social intervention in the families of schizophrenic patients. *British Journal of Psychiatry*, **141**, 121–134.

Leff, J., Kuipers, L., Berkowitz, R., *et al* (1985) A controlled trial of social intervention in the families of schizophrenic patients: two year follow-up. *British Journal of Psychiatry*, **146**, 594–600.

Leff, J., Berkowitz, R., Shavit, N., *et al* (1989) A trial of family therapy v. a relatives group for schizophrenia. *British Journal of Psychiatry*, **154**, 58–66.

Leff, J., Berkowitz, R., Shavit, N., *et al* (1990) A trial of family therapy versus a relatives' group for schizophrenia. Two-year follow-up. *British Journal of Psychiatry*, **157**, 571–577.

LeGrange, D., Eisler, I., Dare, C., *et al* (1992) Evaluation of family therapy in anorexia nervosa: a pilot study. *International Journal of Eating Disorders*, **12**, 347–357.

Lidz, T., Cornelison, A. R., Fleck, S., *et al* (1957) The intrafamilial environment of the schizophrenic patient. II. Marital schism and marital skew. *American Journal of Psychiatry*, **114**, 241–248.

Littlewood, R. (1988) From vice to madness: the semantics of naturalistic and personalistic understandings in Trinidadian local medicine. *Social Science and Medicine*, **27**, 129–148.

Lloyd, T., Kennedy, N., Fearon, P. *et al* (2005) Incidence of bipolar affective disorder in three UK cities: Results from the AESOP study. *British Journal of Psychiatry*, **186**, 126–131.

Mallett, R., Leff, J., Bhugra, D., *et al* (2002) Social environment, ethnicity and schizophrenia: A case control study. *Social Psychiatry and Psychiatric Epidemiology*, **37**, 329–335.

Miklowitz, D. J., Goldstein, M. J., Nuechterlein, K. H., *et al* (1988) Family factors and the course of bipolar affective disorder. *Archives of General Psychiatry*, **45**, 225–231.

Morgan, K. (2003) Insight and psychosis: an investigation of social, psychological and biological factors. Unpublished PhD thesis. Kings College London, University of London.

National Schizophrenia Fellowship (2000) *A Question of Choice*. London: National Schizoprenia Fellowship.

Selvini Palazzoli, M., Boscolo, L., Cecchin, G., *et al* (1978) *Paradox and Counterparadox. A New Model in the Therapy of Schizophrenic Transactions*. New York: Jason Aaronson.

Sharan, S. N. (1966) Family interactions with schizophrenics and their siblings. *Journal of Abnormal Psychology*, **71**, 345–353.

Singleton, N., Maury, N. A., Courie, A., *et al* (2002) *Mental Health of Carers*. London: The Stationery Office.

Swartz, L. (1998) *Culture and Mental Health: A Southern African View*, pp. 84–94. Oxford: Oxford University Press.

Taylor, P. J. & Gunn, J. (1999) Homicides by people with mental illness: myth and reality. *British Journal of Psychiatry*, **174**, 9–14.

Willetts, L. E. & Leff, J. (1997) Expressed emotion and schizophrenia: the efficacy of a staff training programme. *Journal of Advanced Nursing*, **26**, 1125–1133.

Willetts, L. E. & Leff, J. (2003) Improving the knowledge and skills of psychiatric nurses: efficacy of a staff training programme. *Journal of Advanced Nursing*, **42**, 237–243.

Wolff, G., Pathare, S., Craig, T., *et al* (1996) Community knowledge of mental illness and reaction to mentally ill people. *British Journal of Psychiatry*, **168**, 191–198.

Wynne, L. C., Ryckoff, I., Day, J., *et al* (1958) Pseudo-mutuality in the family relations of schizophrenics. *Psychiatry*, **21**, 205–220.

Index

Complied by Caroline Sheard

African culture 9–19
African–Caribbean culture 5–14
alcohol use and abuse 10, 11, 12, 13
antipsychotic medication
    depot injections 15–16, 17
    negative attitudes to 15, 17, 18
    side-effects 15–16, 20
anxiety in carers 7
auditory hallucinations 9, 11, 12, 26

Brixton riots 6

cannabis 5, 7, 8
carer
    death of 40–3
    depression / anxiety 7
    exploitative 91–3
    father as 54–9
    groups 26, 27–8
    mental illness 43–7
    of more than one person 39, 50–4
    overinvolved 11, 12, 22, 44, 53, 61, 62, 73
    patients as 39, 40–3, 47–50
    unsupportive 86–90
children, consideration in treatment plan
    16, 17–18
cognitive–behavioural therapy 38, 45
communication and confidentiality 39
community mental health team 2
confidentiality 77–8
    and communication 39
cultural differences 4–19, 43–7

day centre 8
delusions 35, 37, 38, 44–5, 47
depression in carers 7
diabetes 20, 21–5
dual diagnosis 12

early intervention, benefits of 35
eating disorders 20, 65–72

emotion
    expressed 82
    unexpressed 80–1
emotional divorce 66, 71
evangelical church 6, 7

families
    dysfunctional 77–85
    extended 50–4
    more than one member with psychotic
        illness 39–63
    parental separation or mutual animosity
        64–76
    unsupportive 86–90

grief 40–3
guilt 86–90

hallucinations, auditory 9, 11, 12, 26
hearing impairment 20–1, 25–8, 48
hostel staff overinvolvement 33, 34

India 18–19
infidelity 15, 16
insight 13
institutionalisation 36

learning disability 20, 22–5, 28–38

marital schism 64
marital skew 64
migrants 4–19
mourning 40–3

oculogyric crisis 15
Outsider Art 82
overinvolvement
    by carers 11, 12, 22, 44, 53, 61, 62, 73
    by hostel staff 33, 34

paradoxical intervention 58–9

paranoia and hearing impairment 26
parents
    mutual animosity 64–76
    pseudo-mutuality 79–80
    separation 64–5, 72–6
physical abuse 10, 11, 12
physical illness 20–38, 86–90
pregnancy, illegitimate 9, 11
pseudo-mutuality 79–80
puerperal psychosis 9

racism 5
    institutional 6
rape 86–90
Rastafarian religion 5–6, 7
referral, resistance to 43
relatives with psychotic illness 39–63
role-play 3

sealing over 13
self-esteem 42
sexual abuse 9–14, 86
    delusions of 77–8

slavery 11
social networks 26
spiritual healing 17, 18–19, 21
stigma 78
studiation 10
survivor guilt 62

therapists
    disagreement between 80–1
    support group 94–5
traditional healers 17, 18–19
trauma, unresolved 86–90
twins 59–63

unemployment 6
unresolved past trauma 86–90

violence 36, 38
visual impairment 20–1

weight gain associated with antipsychotic
    use 20